Our Last Promise

To Bill Austin,

It was through your
class that I truly recognized
my love of writing.

All the best!

Kevin

Our Last Promise

A Father and Son's Journey of Hope

Kevin J. Murphy

BLUE HUDSON PUBLISHING

Forest Hills, NY

www.bluehudson.com

© Copyright 2004 Kevin J. Murphy

Blue Hudson Publishing
72-11 Austin Street #190
Forest Hills, NY 11375
Web: http://www.bluehudson.com

ISBN: 0-9721525-4-7
LCCN: 2003092477
First printing 2003. Printed and bound in the United States of America.
All rights reserved.

10 9 8 7 6 5 4 3 2

* The names of all doctors in this book have been changed

ATTENTION ORGANIZATIONS AND GROUPS: Quality discounts
are available for multiple orders of this book. Fundraising copies are also
available for charitable organizations. For information, please contact Blue
Hudson Publishing, 72-11 Austin Street #190, Forest Hills, NY 11375
or sales@bluehudson.com

FOR NORMAL BOOK ORDERS CALL 1-800-781-7595

For everyone who has lost a parent

Acknowledgements

There are a number of people who are important to me that I would like to recognize at the outset of this book.

Mom, I can never repay you for all you have done for me in my life, I can only thank you. You have been a wonderful influence. Thank you for allowing me to take our private moments and share them so that they may help others.

Also thanks to Danny, Sharon, Patrick, and Dianne, for your support and encouragement; Jamie, Benjamin, Daniel, and Michael, as it is through watching you guys that I could relive my childhood; my grandparents for sharing stories from the early days, I'm glad that I took the time to ask when I had the chance; Aunt Jean, Uncle Joe, and Uncle Walter, for your wonderful influences, and for going to keep my father company in heaven; Bruce and Mary Ellen Littmann, for being good friends; Bill Austin, I will never forget that you gave me the inspiration to begin this project; Tracy Meehan, Patti Meehan, Paul Polisciano, Joe Moffa, and John Hetrick, for support and encouragement; Tracy Riva for professional help; Charmaine Alleyne, for being a loving friend and for always having faith in my ability.

Contents

PROLOGUE **Fitting In** 1

ONE **Dad Has Cancer** 5

TWO **Five Years Old** 23

THREE **Should We Talk About It?** 31

FOUR **Seven Years Old** 47

FIVE **Chemotherapy, Radiation, and Prayer** 53

SIX **Nine Years Old** 69

SEVEN **Time is Torture** 75

EIGHT **Eleven Years Old** 85

NINE **Three Squeezes** 93

TEN **Changing Attitudes** 113

ELEVEN **Red Sweatpants** 117

TWELVE **Teenage Years** 137

THIRTEEN **A Sigh of Relief** 143

FOURTEEN **Becoming an Adult** 155

FIFTEEN **There Was No Parachute** 163

EPILOGUE **Our Last Promise** 189

Between grief and nothing I choose grief
—*William Faulkner, The Wild Palms*

Fitting In

The family has decided on pizza for dinner. I am seven years old. Danny, Sharon, and Patrick are all well into their teens.

Nothing I can do is of any use to the family. I can't make money, I can't drive, and I don't even understand most of their grown-up conversations.

I hear Dad yelling from the next room.

"Kev! Come on, let's go get the pizzas! I could really use your help! I have a special job for you. I don't think anybody else can do it."

I like the idea of being able to help. "What kind of job?" I ask.

"Something special! I'll show you when we get there!"

We drive a little while until we reach Brother Bruno's. Dad carries the pies to the car and tells me "You get in first!"

He takes out the blanket he keeps in the trunk, puts it on my legs, and puts the hot pizzas gently on top of it. He goes to the other side and puts the keys in to start the car and tells me about my job.

"*Kev, your job is 'official pizza holder'.*"

Oh, great, a stupid job. Anyone can do that. Nobody needs a pizza holder. "*That's not an important job, Dad!*"

"*Oh no? You remember a few weeks ago when the cheese was stuck to the top of the box?*" *he asks me.*

I nod my head.

"*Well, there was no pizza holder that time. It's an important job. And not just anyone can do it well.*"

I see that he is right. I listen really hard to what he says next.

"*You need to turn the pizzas when the car turns,*" *he tells me.*

I have never heard of this before, but of course there are a lot of things I don't know about.

"*And if we go uphill,*" *he adds,* "*tilt the box the opposite way, with the same degree the car tilts in order to keep it level.*"

"*What's a degree?*"

He laughs. I'm not sure what he's laughing about. Soon he stops laughing.

"*It's a measurement, like an inch. Just do your best, I have faith in you.*"

I feel nervy as we drive home 'cause Bakertown Road has a few bumps on it that might cause the cheese to move.

"*Slow down for the bumps Dad, I don't want the cheese to move!*"

"*Okay!*"

I tilt the pizzas as we climb up the hill on Seven Springs Road. Not being sure what a degree is, I hope I'm tilting them enough.

When we get home Dad puts the pizza boxes on the kitchen table and opens them slowly. He looks from the boxes to me sev-

eral times. I wait to find out if our dinner is okay. I'm kinda jumpy inside. I hope I did a good job.

"Look at that, cheese right there on top of the tomato sauce! Looks like we've found a good job for you, Kev. Thanks for your help!"

I smile ear-to-ear as Mom hands me a paper plate and my brothers and sister come into the kitchen for their slices. Let them have their grown-up conversations. If it weren't for me they couldn't enjoy their pizza. I wonder if they realize how important I am to the family.

ONE

Dad Has Cancer

It was almost midnight. Business at Aer Lingus Cargo was slow and my shift was nearly over, so the guys drew cards in the office to see who would stay to punch the time cards at 12:45. Gabe pulled the loser—four of clubs—and I headed to the locker room to change out of my dirt-soiled clothes. As I was peeling my shirt off my back, I remembered that my father had been to see another doctor that day.

Dad had been feeling bad for more than a month. Since late August, he had seen several doctors, none of whom could determine the cause of his weight loss, weakness, and lack of appetite. His original blood work showed only a slight case of anemia, and even that showed improvement with a follow-up visit. According to the doctors, Dad was healthy. Then he began experiencing chest pain.

Dr. Corning, a cardiologist he knew from six years previous, ordered an echocardiogram, and determined that there was nothing to be concerned about. But Dad continued to feel poorly.

I walked back to the office and checked the clock. 11:58. No doubt Mom and Dad were still awake, relaxing in their reclining chairs watching *The Honeymooners* or some other sitcom rerun.

I dialed the telephone. Mom picked up on the second ring:

"Hello."

"Hi, Mom. You sound like you're on the other line."

"No, I'm just sitting here with your father." Her speech was soft and unbroken, yet her voice possessed an urgency I was not used to. She sounded like a mother who was waiting up for her daughter to return from a first date. I could tell she wasn't ready for sleep.

I was standing up, keys in my hand. My mind was focused on my comfortable bed in my studio apartment, and on waking up for my eight o'clock Economics 101 class the next morning.

"Listen, Mom, I'm on my way out the door," I told her. "I just wanted to know if the doctor said anything today."

"He did. They found a tumor, Kev."

Everything fell silent.

My heart sank.

My world stopped.

A tumor? As in cancer? Fear ripped through my body like a jolt of lightning, supplanting my earlier impatience. I was engulfed in blackness, darkness, the fear of the unknown. Tumors were bad. There was no such thing as a good tumor.

Richie Fabian, Aunt Jean Cronin, my schoolmates Jesse O'Reilly and Kerry O'Donnel came to mind. Cancer had taken them all. I struggled to remember Jesse's face, but I couldn't. I couldn't picture any of them. All I could envision was a red-tailed devil, holding my world in his palm.

"A tumor?" I repeated to Mom.

She was silent, but I could hear the vibration and the whisk of the air as she nodded her head on the other side of the line.

"Mom, hold on one second, okay?"

I removed the phone from my ear and stared at it. Had I dialed the wrong number? Was this the Murphy residence? Was this the right Mom? Surely there was some mistake. These things happen to *other* people. They don't happen to us.

I looked across the room and saw Gabe relaxing comfortably in a chair reading *The Irish Times.* How could he be reading at a time like this?

"Gabe, you go home, I'll punch everyone out," I insisted.

"Are ya shur?" he asked in his Donegal brogue.

"Yeah, go ahead. I'm gonna be a while on the phone."

"Alr-right then Murrrf, have a good nate."

A good night? How could I manage that? Didn't he know about the devil's grasp on the world?

I dropped my keys on the desk and reached for the nearest chair to sit on as Gabe disappeared through the door. I came back to the phone, softer this time, a bit frightened, and without so much confidence.

"Mom, you there?"

"I'm still here."

"What do you mean a tumor?"

"There's a growth in the esophagus. It looks like that's the cause of the problems he's been having. They can't tell us much else yet. They don't know for sure if it's cancerous or not. We have to go for a biopsy on Tuesday."

I grabbed a pen and a notepad as if I thought I was going to need to write something down. I drew a circle on the pad and began retracing it.

"How did it get there?" my numb lips asked.

"They don't know for sure."

I suddenly remembered my father's smoking habit, a habit he had kicked six years earlier as part of his dedication to a healthier lifestyle. My eyes focused on the clock—now past midnight—while I continued retracing the circle on the notepad, over and over.

I wanted more answers. I wanted immediate results, the kind you get with fast-food, e-mail, and digital cameras. I wanted someone to tell me that everything would turn out all right. Would someone please tell me that? Tell me that Dad will see me graduate from college, see me buy my first sports car. Tell me quickly that he will know my children, that he will give them dollar bills to throw into the church collection basket, that he will teach them about model trains at Christmastime.

"So what happens now, Mom? Will it get worse?" I asked her as if she should know the answer. "How do they treat it?"

"These are all questions we're asking too," she told me. "We don't know much more than you do. We have to wait until we go for the biopsy on Tuesday. We're just hoping that it's not cancerous. We'll have to say some prayers."

Silence.

Nobody speaks for a moment.

"Wow," I said. It was all I could think of.

"Want to talk to Dad?" Mom asked.

"Yeah, okay."

The security guard walked through the door. He normally stayed overnight until the morning shift came in.

"How you doin' Kevin?"

"Hey Scott," I said without much interest, hoping he would take a hint that I wanted to be alone. He walked past me and out to the warehouse as Dad came to the phone. I looked down at the notepad. The circle was now dark blue, deeply embossed into the page.

"Hello."

"Hi, Dad. What's all this stuff Mom's telling me about?"

I was hoping he would tell me that it wasn't true, that Mom was confused. Maybe they had been out all night at a party and she had a few drinks. Maybe she was talking about someone else, a distant friend from another state whom I barely knew. Or maybe he could at least tell me that it wasn't very serious, and that it'll just go away soon enough. But he couldn't.

"Some news, hah?" he said like a man trying to take it all in stride.

"Well...h...how do you feel?"

"At least they finally found something," he said with a mixed tone of relief and disappointment. "I was beginning to think I was crazy. Nobody could find anything wrong with me. So on one hand I'm relieved. On the other hand I'm concerned."

"You go back Tuesday?"

"Yeah, then it's two more days to find out the results. This will be a different doctor. He's called a...gastroenterologist."

"Wow," I mumbled in a low disappointed voice. I didn't know what else to say.

Dad took over. "I don't know what to tell you, Kev. We don't have all the pieces to the puzzle yet. Let's see what happens. We'll try to keep a positive attitude."

I drew an X across the circle and put the pen down, then unconsciously began typing letters on the computer screen in front of me.

"Gastroenterologist," he repeated to me. "That's enough to scare me on its own. How do they come up with the names for these specialists?" he asked with a faint chuckle.

It seemed he was hoping to lighten the subject a little. I imagined he was sick of thinking about the whole thing, the seriousness of it. It was a shock to his mind, a shock he had dealt with for the whole day already. His whole life was about to change. He wanted me to tell him a joke, anything to bring his mind some relief, even if for just a moment.

"Gastro-...what?" I played back at him.

"-enterologist. Sounds like he has *some* collection of tools. I hope he doesn't use them all on me," he said, again with a faint chuckle.

"Maybe he'll only use a few," I told him.

"Yeah, I'll tell him that we Irish don't make very good guinea pigs. Hopefully he'll take it easy on me."

"Let's hope so," I said, allowing myself a brief smile.

"Well, we'll all say a few prayers and hopefully everything will turn out okay. Right?"

Dad's positive attitude, along with the thought that prayers would help, brought me a very small measure of ease. But which prayers? Did I know the right ones? What prayers do you say for tumors, for cancer?

"Yeah, okay," I told Dad as I looked at the computer screen:

jjjjjffmmkkkeffkfkfkfkfkmffffffmfmmmmkmkmkmkmkmk.

"So, you have a racquetball tournament this weekend?" he asked.

"Yeah, in New Jersey."

"You're not neglecting your studies, are you?"

"No. Don't worry, you know us young people, we can do anything. You just take care of yourself right now, Dad."

"Okay. So I'll talk to you in a few days, then?"

"Yes."

"Say a couple of prayers, will you? And good luck this weekend."

"Thanks, Dad. I'll say some prayers."

I went home and prayed. I prayed that Tuesday would come quickly and bring better news. I prayed that the tumor would not be cancerous. I told God I was sorry for taking my family's health for granted. I told Him I wished I had been nicer to Jesse in school when he had cancer. I told Him I would do a lot of things different from now on. And I prayed that my father would not join the list of people who died from cancer.

• • •

Finding out that a parent has a potentially fatal disease is shocking, no matter what your age. For me, I was just past childhood and a young adult. I was independent, yes, but not completely removed from my parents' influences. Though I was starting to discover adult life, I still went to my parents when I needed help, or when I wanted recognition or approval for doing something good.

More importantly, I was at a point in my life where I had just begun to appreciate my father for who he was and what he had done for me in my life. I was still trying to make up for the things I had taken for granted as a kid.

Throughout my childhood, I felt that my father and I had a normal relationship. He was okay, I thought, but nothing special. As a youngster, I assumed all Dads were pretty much alike, that they were interchangeable. Being a Dad was a job, just like flipping burgers at McDonald's. And all McDonald's hamburgers came out the same, no matter who was flipping them. Fathers had to love their kids. They had to show up at all the little league games after a hard day at work, unfastening their top buttons and tucking their ties inside their shirt pockets as they hurried toward the field. They had to go out of their way to buy ice cream on their way home from work on Tuesday nights during the summer.

When I was very young, I knew some Dads who stayed home all day with their kids instead of going to those boring jobs, and they watched cartoons and made funny faces and learned the voices of the cartoon characters. Those were the cool Dads when I was a little boy. My Dad couldn't make those funny noises, and he wasn't home to watch the cartoons with me, so he wasn't as cool.

Yet he was still entertaining at times. He used to come home from work and walk up the stairs and say things like "Fee-Fi-Fo-Fum, I smell the blood of a youngest son," in a spooky voice. He grabbed my nose and put his thumb in between his fingers and pretended he had my nose in his hand.

"That's not my nose!" I would yell to him. Then I'd grab his nose. "Now I've got your nose!"

We had play handcuffs and he let me lock him in them and I pretended to lose the key. We also had a game that we played every night right after I put on my Superman pajamas. He put his hands underneath mine with his fingertips touching my palms and in one move tried to come over the top and slap my knuckles. I had to try to move my hands before he slapped them, but I couldn't move until he moved first and he was much faster than me. But eventually I caught up and mastered the game.

Despite these nice times, he couldn't quite measure up to the Dads that didn't have jobs and drank beers all day and made the cartoon sounds. They were so cool that they even took their kids with them sometimes to smoky poker games and to the local tavern for afternoon beers.

As I got a little older, the cartoon-imitating Dads were no longer the coolest. I fell in love with sports, and the best Dads became the ones who were athletic and strong, the ones who coached baseball teams. But my dad wasn't one of these either. He wasn't athletic.

Not that he didn't try. He installed a basketball hoop and shot baskets with me, but he wasn't a good basketball player. He installed horseshoe pits and invited me to learn the game with him, but that wasn't a real sport. He offered many times to have a baseball catch with me, but I often preferred to throw the ball against the brick wall in front of the house. He'd come home in the afternoon and ask me, "Who won today, you or the wall?"

There were other cool Dads too. Those were the ones who didn't bother their kids with questions about school, homework, and what was new. They didn't yell at their son when he got lost hiking up Schunemunk Mountain with Corey Schneider when he was supposed to be home doing his homework. They didn't punish their son for throwing a rock through a neighbor's window, just because he didn't like another boy. They just let their kids be. But again, my Dad didn't measure up to these standards. He asked to see my homework at nights before I was allowed to play softball up the street. He asked me what I was learning in my math class. He asked me if I had any new friends. He asked me to share with him.

"Nothing new, Dad," I usually told him.

One time in fifth grade he heard me on the phone talking to Charlie O'Dell about the new girl in school and how she was weird because she lived in Alaska and how we were going to tease her. "It may be interesting to learn what it was like to live in Alaska, Kev," he told me. Didn't he understand that she was weird?

Don't get me wrong, I had many good times with my father as a boy. Whenever I needed help with my science projects he had good ideas. He cheered me up when I felt down—like in third grade when I pronounced the name Bach as "BATCH" in front of the entire elementary school audience during the talent show. We went on vacations, went fishing, saw movies, threw boomerangs, flew kites, went camping with the Fabians, and tobogganing in the snow down the Monroe golf course. I watched him sing with a barbershop quartet, he helped me fix my bike. We had barbecues, solved a Rubic's cube, and went to the festivals at Bear Mountain and Sugar Loaf. But I didn't share with him as much as he wanted, and I realize now that I hurt his feelings. I would share much more if I could do it over now. But you don't get to do it over; you just get to remember what happened. And you try not to regret, knowing that you were just a little boy at the time—with normal little-boy eyes and little-boy reactions.

In my mid-teens, the definition of a cool Dad changed once again. And once again, my Dad didn't fit in. The cool Dads were the ones that let you drink beer, let you have parties at the house, let you stay out as late as you wanted and not even come home at all some nights. My father was nothing like that. We got into arguments about right and wrong, about what I should and shouldn't be allowed to do, and about the world and what was happening in it. He didn't seem to know much about what was important in life and what went on in the real world—and of course, I had already figured it all out as a teenager.

As I continued to envy the cool Dads of my times and wish that I had one, I missed out on all the wonderful things about my father. They slipped right past me. He tried to stop me sometimes and make me see them, but I didn't have time. There were other things I needed to do.

Strangely enough, it was in Texas, fifteen hundred miles away from Dad—where he couldn't have the same daily influences on me that he did back home—that my metamorphosis took place.

At the age of eighteen I left college after my first semester because I decided that I wanted to get my flying certificates. I had recently received my private pilot's license and decided on a school in Texas to continue my studies in this area, get my instrument rating, commercial license, and flight instructor certificate. Then I would be able to give flight instruction while going to school and build up my flight hours.

I left for Dallas in early February of that year and did not return home again until November. I usually called home on Sunday nights. Mom normally answered the phone and I talked to her first.

"Are you getting enough to eat?" she'd ask.

"Yes, Mom"

"Do you have clean sheets?"

"I washed yesterday."

"Are you staying out of trouble?"

"Of course I am."

"Do you miss me?"

"Oh, Mom. I miss you very much."

And I did miss her. She was always nice. She was a kind person, and more importantly when I was a kid, she didn't ask me the tough questions. She didn't come down hard on me when I did something wrong. Those things were Dad's job. She supported him, yes, but as a kid I naively thought she was secretly against these disciplines.

After our conversation she would give the phone to Dad. If they had company, as they often did on a Sunday night, Mom would tell me he was excusing himself from the company to go into his room to talk with privacy. At first I thought this meant lectures about things like making sure I was on my best behavior, about how much money they were investing in me, and to make sure I was "on the ball".

But to my surprise, these lectures never came. Instead he asked me about the weather, the people, the differences between New York and Texas. He asked how the flying was going, reminded me not to forget to have fun, and told me to call if I ever needed anything, and to call if I just wanted someone to talk to.

Other than a few dollars here and there, I never called to ask for anything, yet I called often just to talk, and I began to feel a real fondness for my father.

"You should see the clouds outside today," I told Dad one day. "I've been watching them build throughout the day, they're gonna explode into a storm in a little while."

"I like thunderstorms, they're very intense," he told me.

"Really? I didn't know that about you!"

"Yeah, sometimes I like to grab a beer and watch the storm from the front porch," he said.

"You do? I never noticed!"

"That's because you always had your own things going on!" he laughed. "But I think there's nothing quite like an intense storm and a cold beer on a warm day."

"Wow, that's exactly what I like! I mean, I would if I were old enough to drink."

He laughed. "Yeah, I know what you mean."

Our conversations got longer as the weeks went on. Normally I told him about how the flying was going and different stories about being up in the air. I told him about the differences in the food, the roads, the dress, the lifestyle of Texas. I told him about rodeos, town dances, and country music. At some point I started asking him what he did each week, and he told me about his new lawnmower, the books he was reading, and his favorite hobby, woodcarving. He was into carving birds and falcons at that time. He told me about what he and Mom did on weekends, and the expeditions he went on with Mr. Littmann.

When I wasn't talking to him I found myself thinking about him often during the week. I thought about how much his input helped me in my decisions about what to do after high school, decisions like joining the navy or going to college and joining ROTC. I wondered what he was doing each day, if he was carving something new—and what advice he would give me if he were here.

And I realized that I missed him. I had always known my father, the parent. I had to move fifteen hundred miles away to appreciate my father, the man. I learned that he was a kind person, that he adored my mother, and that he had a lot of interests and talents. I understood now that he'd made sacrifices for me, and whether I appreciated them or not, he would never regret making them. For the first time in my life the facts that had always been in front of me came into focus. My father was not just a man named John whom God happened to give me a genetic link to, but instead, was quite an extraordinary person; a person others respected; a man who loved his wife and family unconditionally; a person who understood that people sometimes make mistakes. He was talented, unique in character, and someone who didn't need lots of recognition and fanfare to be satisfied with his own accomplishments. More than that, I realized that the things I knew and many of the ways I behaved had been learned from him, even though I didn't recognize that at the time.

And, at some point during my ten months in a Dallas suburb, I realized that real heroes don't always wear capes, hit home runs, or slam-dunk basketballs. Sometimes they're right in front of us every day, doing the very things we come to expect and too often take for granted.

• • •

The weekend after finding out about the tumor, I played in a racquetball tournament in New Jersey, and I brought a book with me about tumors and cancer that I checked out of the college library.

I read the book in between my matches, amidst the echoing of racquetballs being pounded on the court and the boisterous players complaining to referees. The book told me about how tumors form because cells become abnormal, divide, reproduce in the body and cluster together. It talked about benign tumors, malignant tumors, radiation, chemotherapy, and metastasis.

I thumbed through the pages. Was this it? Where was the solution? Where was the outcome? I desperately shuffled through chapters, looking for one that would cover *my* family's situation, one entitled "Your Dad's Tumor". I hoped the chapter would be short, painless, and have a happy ending. I envisioned a picture of my father standing triumphant over the disease on page four.

But, as the scent of sports cream whisked through the air, I realized there was no such chapter. I kept reading, hoping to find some hint, somewhere, of what was going to happen, how he would be treated, or what prayers I should say.

But I found nothing in the book to ease my mind. I only found more questions.

That night I said prayers, beginning with a simple talk with God. *God, as you know, Dad is having some health problems. Please let him come through it okay. He's a good person, and he means a lot to me. Please don't let him have any pain or have to have any operations. Please just let everything be okay.*

Then I said an *Our Father*, a *Hail Mary*, and at the end, I smiled, because it made me feel a little better. And that's what the prayers were all about. God wasn't in need of my prayers, and neither was Dad. But I was in need of saying them. They made me feel better.

• • •

Tuesday arrived like a school bus when you don't have your homework done. I didn't want it to come.

The gastroenterologist performed an endoscopy of Dad's throat. Though the official results would not be known for two days, the doctor told my parents, "I've seen enough to be certain that it is cancer".

In the house where I grew up, cursing was discouraged. Yet my mother summed up her thoughts that evening with characteristic serenity. She sat on the reclining chair and softly said, "Oh, shit".

"That's just what I was thinking," Dad replied.

Somehow I still held out hope that the doctor was wrong. It can't be cancer. It was all happening so quick. He just has a little problem with his appetite. Make him eat some food, doctors, you'll see.

But on Thursday, when the official results confirmed the esophageal cancer, I had to acknowledge the reality of the situation.

The tumor, lodged at the base of Dad's esophagus, was seven inches long and about the size of a silver dollar in diameter. It appeared to be leaning on the left lung, although the doctors were not completely sure. The plan was to begin treating the disease within two weeks. Dad would stay in the hospital for four days of chemotherapy, simultaneously beginning fifteen consecutive days of radiation treatments. Shortly after that time, he would go back into the hospital for four more days of chemotherapy. The treatment was designed to stop the spread of the cancer and to shrink the tumor to make for an easier surgical removal.

The surgery would be a risk. Six years earlier, Dad had double bypass surgery and any surgery now would be dangerous. I didn't comprehend the gravity of the situation during his heart condition. I went to the hospital to donate blood for him, but I was just starting eleventh grade and was distracted by the wondrous feelings I was having over my first "true love". But he came through the surgery in good shape.

The condition of Dad's heart was the second catalyst to his quitting smoking. When his first grandchild, Jamie, arrived two years earlier, he had cut down on cigarettes and wouldn't light up in the house or anywhere near Jamie. He didn't want to subject his newfound love to any harmful smoke. She was much too important to him. Then, after the heart surgery, he never smoked another cigarette. But that was about the only thing his heart condition put an end to, although Mom, Grandma, and even his kids often tried to discourage him from shoveling snow and other strenuous tasks.

The surgery to remove the tumor would be risky due to his heart condition. It would be supervised by the cardiologist, Dr. Corning. The surgery would take place a couple of weeks after the radiation and chemotherapy treatments ended.

The night the cancer was confirmed I prayed again, harder this time. *Bad news, God. It looks like we're at the beginning of a tough ordeal. What do we do now? Please help us. We need help.*

I hoped God would show us a plan. The doctors had a plan, yes. But they didn't have a solution. And that's what cancer is like. It's like someone throws you out of an airplane and gives you a backpack and tells you there *might* be a parachute inside. You fall, struggling against the wind to strap the backpack on, hoping that when you pull the chord, there will be a parachute and it will work.

TWO

◦——//——◦

Five Years Old

Mom seems to be upset. She tells Dad on the phone "The mortgage is too high, I just broke a chair, and I don't know where Danny and Patrick are!"

She doesn't ask me to help 'cause I'm only five and Danny and Patrick are much taller than me. I'm probably too short to reach the mortgage without standing on the chair and now the chair is broked. I can see why she's so upset.

A little while later she says, "We're going to meet Dad where he goes fishing" and tells me, "Get ready!".

"Okey-dokey," I tell her.

Soon we're in the car and drive for a little while until we see Dad's car on the side of the road and we pull up beside it and I follow Mom down a hill and we look for Dad. I've never been here before but Mom says, "It's called Woodbury Creep".

Mom says Dad comes here one or two times each week after work during the summer and I ask "Does he really like to fish so much?" but she tells me he comes here to dream a little and to do something with Stress and I am confused. I'm not sure who Stress is unless he's one of my uncles that live on Long Island who we don't see very often and I don't think Dad is silly enough to fall asleep and have dreams at the fishing stream. I don't think Mom understands why he comes here, but surely she'll figure it out when she sees him with the fishing pole.

The stream is really nice. There are lots of big rocks and the water makes a neat sound when it hits them. It's not very deep and Mom and Dad let me walk on the rocks. I hop from one rock to the next and sometimes I reach all the way to the other side without touching the water and that's really cool!

Mom takes her shoes off and sits on the edge of the stream under a tree and dips her feet in the water while Dad fishes from a big rock in the center of the stream. Mom talks about the mortgage again and a few things I don't understand about and Dad listens as he moves his wrist back and forth and the fishing line follows his motion. He tells me "We're fishing for trout" and says, "We use flies to try to catch them".

Trout is a kind of fish but I don't understand how something that swims below the water thinks it's gonna eat something that flies above the ground. Each time he drags the line back in I look for the trout but I never see one and I wonder what they look like and how big they are and why they like flies.

When Mom's done talking she cries and Dad asks me "You wanna try it?" and gives me a quick lesson on how to hold the rod. He says, "Most people call it a pole" but tells me, "It's proper to call it a rod".

Dad goes over to Mom and sits in the shade with his arm around her and I grip the rod with two hands and wait for a fish that likes flies. I can't hear what they are talking about, but I'm sure it's about me and what a good fisherman I am.

• • •

We're standing in line at Woodbury town hall on Election Day. Although I'm not sure exactly what Election Day really is I know that one-by-one people are disappearing into a booth only to reappear a minute later. It seems like the magic show at the circus Mom and Dad took me to last year, 'cept there's no magician and I don't understand the tricks.

Another person is coming out now; same clothes she had on going in, still two arms, legs, and a serious look. I haven't seen anyone laughing when they come out. What happens in there?

I remember this place from last year; I stood with Mom while Dad voted and with Dad while Mom voted. Maybe if I bug Dad a little he'll offer to let me go into the booth with him.

I tug on his coat and he looks down at me.

"Dad, what happens when you go into the booth?"

"Well, first you pull the curtain, then you push levers for who you want to vote for, then you lock it in, and then you pull the curtain to come out."

"Isn't there someone in there who asks who you want to vote for?"

He starts laughing. I don't know why he is laughing. Soon he stops laughing.

He bends his knees and brings himself down to my height. "No, it's not like that," he says. "Why don't you come in with me and I'll show you."

"Yep, okay."

As the moment nears I am a little scared. I haven't seen any other kids go in with their parents. I hear you have to be an adult to vote, I hope whatever's in there doesn't know I'm not an adult. I hope it doesn't eat kids.

"Our turn, Kev," he tells me.

"Are you sure it's okay, Dad? I don't think I want to go."

"Look, there's nothing to be scared of, I promise. It'll be a good experience for you." He bends down again and puts his hand on my shoulder. "Nothing bad will happen, I promise you. Okay?"

"Okey-dokey."

He takes my hand and we walk into the booth. The curtain closes behind us but there is a light in the booth. Lots of levers, but nobody in here to ask who we are voting for. It's just me and Dad. It's very small in here.

Dad begins to push levers with so much ease. I can tell he's very good at it. He tells me that one of the levers lets you vote for a whole bunch of people at one time, but he doesn't use that one.

"This one is for the local judge," he says. "I think your friend's father is running."

I see a button that says Levinson. I wonder if it's really Josh's Dad.

"Can we vote for him?" I ask.

"Yeah, I was going to," he tells me. "You want to push the button?"

I'm scared. "No, you do it," I tell him.

"C'mon, you'll be the first little kid to vote!" he says.

A feeling of power comes over me. I push the lever for Levinson. Later I learn that he wins. I think it's probably because of me.

We open the curtain. I remember to put on my serious look. I wonder if others are watching me.

•　•　•

Mom is in front of me as we stand in the checkout line at Jamesway.

"Can we get this, Mom?"

I hold up a small box of green chewable candy. They look like tic-tacs, only a little bigger.

"Kevin, I think you already have enough candy at home."

"Please, Mom?" I beg her. She usually buys me anything I want.

"C'mon, put it back. You don't need those. You have more candy than any kid on the block."

"Ooo-keeey-dooooo-keey."

But these candies are unlike any I've ever seen before. They have a bright shine to them and I can only imagine what they must taste like. I have to have them.

Mom isn't watching carefully, she is handing the clerk her stuff. I know she won't buy the greens and nobody is watching me. I think about the shine of the greens and the taste that must follow. I must have them. I put them in my pocket and don't say a word!

We drive home and I look for a good hiding spot for the greens. Underneath my pillow is the best spot.

Mom comes to tuck me in for bed and I get scared as she approaches the bed. Will she know? Will she find the candy? Will she ask if I took them?

What do I do?

She starts to ask me questions.

"Did you say your praye..."

"Yep."

"Brush your tee..."

"Yep."

"Say good-night to your fath..."

"Yep."

"What's wrong? Why are you in such a hurry? You act like there's something wrong."

"What could be wrong? You think I'm hiding something? I'm not! There's nothing here, let's just shut the lights out and go to bed."

I point at the lights. I hold my pillow tightly. My lips are shaking.

"Why are you talking to me like that? And what are you hiding under your pillow?"

"Nothing."

"Nothing? Let me see this nothing."

"It's nothing, I promise."

She lifts me up, pillow and all, and picks up the candy that was underneath.

"What's this, Kevin?"

"I don't know," I tell her, still holding tightly onto the pillow.

"How did this get under your pillow?"

"I don't know."

"You don't know?"

My lips keep shaking. I can't take it anymore.

"I stole it! I stole it! Okay! Now will you leave me alone?"

Dad comes running into the room when he hears me scream. I hold the pillow tightly against my stomach. There is something dancing around in my stomach now.

"John, he stole these green candies from the store today!" Mom tells Dad.

"What?" he screams. Boy am I gonna get it now. A six-year old thief I am.

Mom gives him the candies. He looks at them and smells them.

"*Kevin, what's this Mom's telling me about these green candies?*"

"*I don't know,*" *I tried again.*

"*I think you do know,*" *he says as he bends over to sit next to Mom on the edge of my bed. I back into the corner of the bed against the wall. My pillow is my only friend now.*

"*Kevin, you can't just take things. It's against the law. More important, it's wrong.*"

"*I know,*" *I tell him.*

"*Well, if you know, then why did you do it?*"

"*Cause they looked good.*"

He shakes his head. "*Lots of things look good, but we can't always have them. It's part of life.*"

Mom moves over a little bit on the bed to give Dad more room on the bed and he gets closer to me. My whole body is bouncing now. Tears are falling down my cheeks.

"*Relax, Kev,*" *he says as he puts his hand on my knee.* "*It's important that you listen to me now.*"

Mom gives me a tissue to wipe my face.

"*If we could all just take what we want, I would have a shiny sports car.*"

"*But they'd catch you,*" *I tell him.*

He shakes his head. "*That's not what stops me from taking it. I don't take it because it's not right. It's not mine. You understand?*"

I nod my head. He takes the pillow away and lifts me out from the corner and puts his arm around my neck.

"*I'm not going to tell you about how angry I am right now. But do you realize you shouldn't take something that belongs to someone else?*"

"*But it wasn't someone else's, Dad, it was the store's,*" *I tell him as I wipe my face.*

"It's still not yours. Whether it's another person's or the store's, it doesn't matter. Isn't that right, hon?" he asks as he turns to Mom.

"That's right. It's not yours," she says.

"You said prayers tonight, right?" he asks me.

I nod.

"What do you think God thinks about you taking these?"

"He's probably mad," I say.

"Well, I don't think God gets mad, but he's certainly disappointed. I know I'm disappointed in you."

"Are you going to punish me?"

A loud breath comes from his nose. "Probably. We'll talk about that tomorrow. But it's not the punishment you should be afraid of. Isn't the disappointment enough? You should be disappointed in yourself."

I nod my head.

"Tomorrow you'll take back the candy with Mom and ask the people at Jamesway to forgive you. In the meantime ask God to forgive you. And I want you to do something good tomorrow to try to make up for today."

The next day we take the candy back and later I invite some of the kids over and we play "The Price is Right" and I give away some of my best toys as prizes. Chris Melcher wins my favorite matchbox car. I hate to lose that car. I hope it makes up for stealing the green candy.

THREE

Should We Talk About It?

The Saturday after learning about the cancer, I drove home to see my parents. Perplexing thoughts raced through my mind on the hour and a half drive to Highland Mills. How should I act? How are children supposed to act when their parents have cancer? Do I ask Dad about it? Do I pretend like nothing has changed? Do I hug him and hold him tight? Do I tell him I love him so much and cry? Or do I try to maintain an easygoing attitude and appear confident that everything will be okay? Do we talk about how I'm doing in school, my racquetball tournaments? Or do we talk about cancer treatments and doctors and such? I thought about all of this on the drive, but came up with only one answer. I didn't know what to do or how to act. It was like I was the prodigal son returning home for the first time in many years.

Mom and Dad were at the top of the stairs when I walked through the front door. As I climbed the stairs, the "don't look" feeling came over me. You know the feeling:

it's the one you get when someone you know has something about him that is different from usual. It happens when you haven't seen someone for a long time, or when a person has a new hairstyle, shaved off his mustache, or has lost a lot of weight. You try to avoid looking directly at them, either because you don't want to stare at the person's change in appearance, or, as in my case that day, because you don't know what to say. It was almost like Dad was a new person, a stranger.

Usually, I was the one with the problem and Dad was the one who helped solve it. He always seemed to be the strongest person on earth. In my mind, nothing bad could ever touch him, and if something tried, he would just swat it away like King Kong did to the airplanes in the movies. Surely he would go through this cancer thing quickly and come out unfazed. After all, there were many cases in which people had survived cancer and led healthy lives. Yes, many people had died from the disease too, but this was my father and it wasn't going to happen to him. I wouldn't even consider that possibility. The doctors knew where the tumor was; they could shrink it, and then remove it. Problem solved. It all seemed so simple in September.

"Hi Kev," Mom said when I was halfway up the stairs. "How are you feeling?"

That's an easy question. It has nothing to do with cancer, diseases, tumors, or illness.

"A little better than last week," I told her. "I think I finally shook my cold, or whatever it was I had."

"I hope you don't have what I have!" Dad interjected.

His words stunned me. I was like a deer caught in the headlights, not knowing which way to move. The deer usually stands still. Did he mean that to be funny? This was a direct question, was it meant to bring about an open acknowledgement of his disease? It made me uncomfortable. Weren't we supposed to pretend nothing was wrong?

I broke a half-smile. "I don't think so, Dad. How are you?" I asked as I reached the top of the stairs.

Before I knew what was happening he grabbed me from the stairs and threw his arms around me and squeezed me tightly. I was stunned again, like I had been hit by flash lightning. I had expected a handshake and a wink. I thought he would pretend everything was okay, that there was no cancer. I put my arms around his waist and hugged him back. He squeezed harder. I clasped my fingers together behind him. Mom watched us. I struggled for a breath. I moved my arms higher up his back and squeezed. I thought about how frightened he must be. How scary it is to have cancer. I couldn't speak. There were no words as powerful as the hug.

"It's good to have you here," Dad said as he continued to embrace me.

"I'm glad I'm here," I said. "We'll get through this," I told him.

"Yeah, I know we will." He pulled back from me and looked into my eyes. His eyes were moist. He winked at me.

"You can beat cancer, Dad. We can beat it together." I was happy to say the word, cancer. It was a difficult word to actually say, much more difficult to say than to write or to think about. But Dad had broken the ice that I needed broken, and I realized that acknowledging the cancer and talking about it were not really "taboo" as I thought they might be.

A new lane opened in our relationship. For the first time in my life Dad very much needed me, as I had needed him many times in the past. If I could have that moment back to do over, I would race up the stairs and be the one to put my arms out first and hug him. I wouldn't need to say anything.

As the day progressed we talked a little about the tumor. He explained how it was blocking his esophagus and that was why he couldn't enjoy food. It was difficult to get the food down his throat and the taste was altered. We discussed the treatment procedure and talked about the various doctors involved. He sounded confident in their approach.

"They're the professionals, Kev," he said. "I think we should trust their judgment."

"Just make sure they know how important you are!" I told him.

He smiled.

"Make sure they know that you have a lot of sculptures left to carve," I said.

"Speaking of carving, I want to show you my horse, it's almost done," he said referring to his carousel wood-carving project.

Woodcarving was his passion. I admired his talent, especially since he had only taken up the hobby six years earlier. He always had a knack for working with wood, whether it was making the best marshmallow sticks when we went camping or making a guitar for my sister, a crib for his grandchildren, or a cribbage table for him and Mom to play cards. But the woodcarving was something more. It was like a second love for him. He seemed at peace when he was alone in the garage with his woodcarving tools and a block of wood.

Each piece he carved contained a little slice of Dad. In some I saw his humor, like the carving of two dogs licking a bottle of beer that had spilled on the floor, and he even made a thin stream of lager-colored glue going from one dog's tongue to the spill. In others I saw his views of life, like the one where he carved four tiny men sitting on mushrooms. They were four men from different walks of life. One was Abe Lincoln, another was a jogger, one looked like Grandpa Murphy and had little polka dots on his tie, and the fourth was a farmer with his hands in his pockets. When I asked Dad about it he told me, "If you go back far enough, Kev, everyone comes from the same mushroom patch".

My favorite carving was of an eagle. It had a five-foot wingspan and was his first major piece. The whole family was astonished at his accomplishment when we saw the finished work. After all these years, a new talent just popping up out of the blue, it was remarkable. "Don't Tread on Me," the red, white, and blue banner across the breast of the eagle read. I asked him how he went about carving something like that and he said to me, "You just take a block of wood and cut out everything that doesn't look like eagle."

He had been working on the miniature carousel horse for a few years, routinely doing a little bit of work, then stopping for months at a time while he studied the intricacies of how to detail the next part.

"I'm just finishing up working on the tail," he told me as we entered the garage to look at the horse.

It was a marvelous piece. About half the size of the

horses you ride on at carousels; the real carousels, the ones with real wooden horses, not the manufactured ones. I took carousels for granted too, but never again. Hard to believe I followed this one from its inception; from a few blocks of wood to a soon-to-be carousel horse prancing in our living room.

"Hey guys!" Mom yelled from upstairs. "Time for dinner!"

I was excited about the prospects of a home cooked meal. I didn't get many good meals in college. Dad rolled his eyes. Dinner was like a necessary evil for him. He had to have some nourishment, but eating was no longer an enjoyable experience. We left the horse in the garage and went upstairs, where some of Dad's finished carvings kept us company during dinner; birds, falcons, geese, ducks, even a duck hunter. Dad wasn't able to eat much dinner. He tried, but had to excuse himself from the table after a little while and go inside.

"After a little while," Mom said to me, "just the sight of food makes him queasy."

Mom went into the living room to sit with Dad while I stayed in the kitchen finishing my pot roast. She didn't like him to feel alone.

I envied the relationship that my parents had together. Love was one thing, but they had something more than that. I admired how they interacted with each other, and how they gave each other the freedom to interact with others. And the caring that they felt for one another, the trust they had in each other. They were soul mates.

There was a time when I came home from college and went out to eat with Mom and Dad at the Black Forest. It was a German restaurant they frequented every couple of weeks together. The host's eyes lit up when she saw them. After we sat down, a waitress from the next room came over to say hello and told our waitress to take good care of us. Even at the end of the meal, when Mom was still eating and Dad and I were finished, Dad wouldn't let the busboy take his plate away because he didn't want Mom to feel like she was eating alone. Mom was a notoriously slow eater and it made her uncomfortable to be the only one left with food at the end of a meal. "I'm still picking on it a little bit," Dad told the young Mexican busboy while pointing at the plate. The kid looked at the mouthful of potatoes left on the plate and scratched his head. Dad then picked up his fork every once in a while and pretended he was still eating while he talked to Mom and I.

While we were waiting for desert I wanted to check the score on a basketball game so I went into the bar and asked the bartender to change the channel. I struck up a conversation with her and when she asked me who I was with, I said, "You must know my parents. They come here all the time."

When I described them she gave me a funny look. "You mean Miriam and John?"

"Yes," I told her.

"I never knew they were married," she said as she shook her head. Then she proceeded to tell me that the way they looked at each other so lovingly and talked to each other so nicely, the way they held each other's hands; she thought they were boyfriend and girlfriend. The romance and love was still there. She told me that they seemed to be on a date whenever she saw them, and she was often tempted to serve them just one glass and two straws.

• • •

Two weekends after learning about the cancer, the entire
Murphy family got together in New Jersey to celebrate my
Grandfather's ninetieth birthday party. My cousin, Amy,
found a Knights of Columbus hall and caterer in Montclair
for a reasonable price.

The family scored perfect attendance; it was the first
time in many years that had happened. There were aunts,
uncles, cousins, and second cousins, forty-three people in
all.

I sat in the back seat of my brother Danny's car on the
way to the party. The invitations said to be there at one
o'clock, and at 1:30 we were surprised to be only the second car in the church parking lot across the street. The
other car was my parents'. My sister Sharon and her kids
rode with them, and my other brother Patrick arrived in
his van a few minutes later. This gave the immediate Murphy
family some time alone before everyone else showed up.
There was a sense of closeness in the family unlike any I
had felt before.

Nobody but us knew about Dad's cancer. Mom and
Dad hadn't told anyone else yet. A week earlier, they had
gone to a wedding attended by most of their good friends
and former neighbors from Queen's Village. They hadn't
mentioned it to anyone there either.

The hall was set up with six tables, each having five to
eight chairs around them. All the food was set up in the
kitchen, buffet style, and coolers with different beers and
sodas and a couple of wines lined one of the walls. In the

middle of the hall was a big collage with pictures from the past, representing the different stages of Grandpa Murphy's ninety years; pictures of him in his army uniform, pictures of him wearing different hats and clothes of the decades past, pictures of him and Grandma smiling with different grandchildren.

In order to limit the shock for a ninety-year-old man, Grandma told Grandpa about the party a few minutes before walking through the door. Nevertheless, when he walked through the door and we yelled "Surprise!" it seemed like he wasn't expecting it.

A local pastor came by to give a special blessing to my grandparents. "May God's love continue to shine on these two wonderful individuals and their great family," he pronounced.

"How many years are you guys married now?" he asked my grandparents informally.

"Sixty-three," Grandpa snapped back at him with pride.

"Well, now I can tell you the secret of marriage," he announced to us all with a serious face, as if he were about to reveal some kind of ancient secret. "It's the first sixty-three years that are the toughest. After that it's all downhill!" Everyone laughed and applauded. It was like we were applauding the lifetime accomplishments of my grandparents.

I found my grandparents very interesting and accomplished in life. Not accomplished in individual achievements, but rather in the way that they seemed to know what was important in life: family, love, happiness. And they passed those things on to all those around them, not by preaching, but by showing, and by letting others join in it with them.

Both of them had come from interesting backgrounds: Grandma grew up in Nanticoke, Pennsylvania, the last of nine children—two of whom died as infants—where she baked pies and desserts in her family's business. Grandpa was orphaned at an early age and spent time in England and Ireland before he immigrated to Canada at the age of eighteen.

The pictures in the collage, especially the older ones, made me and many of my cousins curious, and we surrounded my grandparents at various times to ask them about some of their earlier days.

I came over to them sitting at a table as Grandma was finishing a story. It was something about being detained on her return to the United States from Canada over suspected bootlegging during the prohibition era. I wished I could have heard the whole story. When I reached the table, Julie, Jenny, Mary, and Steve were hysterical at the image of Grandma as an Al Capone-style bootlegger.

"What about you Grandpa, any gangster stories?" my cousin Jenny asked.

"Well, just the time in Chicago. What you guys know as the St. Valentine's Day Massacre."

"Was that near you?" she asked.

"Two minutes before it happened I was on that very block," he said. "I turned the corner and got about two blocks away and heard the gunshots. We didn't know what was happening."

"And you, what do you want to know, Kevin?" Grandma asked as she noticed me standing with one hand in my pocket and the other grasping a cold beer.

"What was your first job?" I asked.

"Oh, that was in the movie theatre," she told me. "The movies of those days didn't have any sound. I played the piano."

"Did you rehearse?" I asked.

"There was nothing to rehearse. Every day it was a different movie. I just watched the movie like everyone else. When the villain appeared I played Dum-De-Dum-Dum. When something funny happened I played the high notes. They didn't pay much but there weren't many jobs for women those days. We weren't even allowed to vote until I moved to New York."

"Is that where you guys met?" my cousin Stephanie interjected as she walked into the mix.

"No, we met at the Horn and Hardet on Broadway. I worked nine to five and Grandpa worked the night shift. Of course we called him Red in those days."

"Red?" Stephanie asked. Not that we thought his hair was always white, but the pictures were black and white so we couldn't tell what color it was.

"Yeah, he had the brightest red hair you'd ever seen. And he came in late every day to work and I had to cover for him all the time and that was how we got to know each other."

"Remember the time I got arrested?" Grandpa interjected.

"Oh, yeah. You make me laugh," she said.

"Arrested?" I asked.

"Yeah, after work I went swimming with a couple of the fellas and I was the last one out. When I came out of the water everyone else had left and they hid my clothes and I couldn't find them. A police officer arrested me for indecent exposure!"

As we all laughed, I broke away from the conversation to get a fresh beer, but each moment there were new people joining in and others leaving. It was like a rotation of listeners.

I started mixing around the room and finding other conversations. I talked to my cousin Mike, who was actively involved with various campaigns. "Are you campaigning for Cuomo this year? You think he's going to win again?" I asked him.

"Mario? Yeah, he's got some great programs going now," Mike said.

Soon Rich and Carol were by us and we talked to them about the excitement of becoming parents for the first time. When I saw Matt, I talked to him about the weather in Texas, because he had spent some time there too. Chris and Julie loved sports, and I had a conversation with them comparing racquetball and tennis.

During all these conversations, I found that I could never get my father out of my mind and was constantly moving my eyes to find his whereabouts and see what he was doing. I saw my cousins Jenny, Pat, Thomas, and Julie talking to him. I saw Rudy, Gerry, and Maureen having conversations with him. Considering Dad was scheduled to begin chemotherapy three days later, he seemed to be in high spirits at the party. Though he wasn't able to have a beer and didn't eat very much, he smiled a lot and seemed comfortable talking to my cousins who approached him throughout the day to have a conversation with their "Uncle John". But his situation had to be paramount on his mind.

At one point during the afternoon I noticed him sitting at one of the tables talking privately to Danny and Dianne. By their body language, I concluded it was a serious conversation and I thought it might be about his condition. If it was, I wanted to be involved, so I went over to join in. When I sat down, even though I didn't say anything, it was as though I had forced myself into the conversation, and I realized they weren't talking about Dad's condition.

While the background had sounds of young kids playing tag and running around the chairs and younger kids crying to their mothers, Dianne told me, "We're talking about adopting a child, Kev. We were just getting Dad's opinion about it."

"Oh, very nice," I said.

Dad gave me a long look, then focused back on Dianne and said "Listen, if you're going to adopt, I urge you to consider an older child."

Though I thought it was a serious statement, Dianne began to laugh and slapped Dad playfully across his chest. "Daaad! Not that old!" she yelled.

Just then he smiled and I realized he had been pointing at me behind my back, as if he wanted to give me up for adoption.

"Hey!" I said. "I'm too old to be adopted. You're stuck with me!"

He reached his hand out to pat my shoulder and laughed. A nice laugh. I hoped to keep hearing that laugh for a long time.

Late in the afternoon, as everyone was saying their good-byes, Mom pulled Grandma aside to tell her the grave news about the cancer. Grandma was silent for a moment, and then she looked into Mom's eyes and said, "If prayers can help, he will get better because we will pray every minute of the day for our son".

Dad and I also didn't speak about the cancer and chemotherapy until we were leaving. But the party was just a distraction from the cancer, and now that the party was over and I was alone with Dad, the reality set in once again.

"Have you thought about what it might be like on Tuesday?" I asked as we were packing the last of the left-over food into the back of his Chevy Blazer.

"Some. The doctors have explained it," he told me as Jamie ran over to him, handed him another toy that needed to be packed into the truck, then darted back inside to finish her good-byes to her generation of cousins.

"How long will it take?"

"I don't really know, Kev. They have to put something called a mediport in my body first to disperse the medicine. I think it may take a while the first day."

"I'll be thinking about you that day," I said. I paused to think about what I must sound like. Just that day, the day he starts the chemotherapy?

"Well, I'm thinking about you every day," I quickly added. "But especially Tuesday."

"I know what you mean." He put his hand on my shoulder as we closed the back window of the truck. "Party was nice, eh?"

"Yeah. Imagine living to be ninety?"

He shook his head. "Not yet. I'm gonna just concentrate on making it to fifty-six right now."

Yes, thinking about ninety is a luxury he can't afford himself right now. What a stupid thing for me to say. Or am I just being over sensitive? Just say what comes to mind, Kev. No regrets.

"You'll make it," I said. "I mean, *we'll* make it. Together."

"Yeah, I think you're right."

It was time to leave. I put my arms out and hugged him. I gave him a long squeeze.

"Good luck this week," I said. "If you're scared, remember we'll all be with you."

FOUR

❧ ⚜ ❧

Seven Years Old

Dad is in the backyard talking to one of the neighbors. There's a chainsaw dangling from his right hand. They're pointing to a tree.

"I think if we don't cut it down now it may fall during the next big storm. I don't want it coming through our bedroom," Dad says.

"I think this is the best angle, John," the neighbor tells him.

I run down the porch steps toward them.

"Don't cut the tree, Dad! Please? I love that tree!"

"It has to come down, Kevin. Would you rather it fell on the house?"

"Yes I would! Besides, it won't fall. I promise!"

He shakes his head and frowns. "Sorry, Kev. It has to come down."

I run back into the house and slam my bedroom door. A little while later there is a knock.

"Hey Kev, I've got something I want to show you outside. It's a surprise!" he says, his clothes covered with sawdust.

"A surprise?"

"Yeah, c'mon!"

I am angry at him for cutting down the tree, but I like the idea of a surprise. I hope it's a good one.

I follow him down the hall and out to the back yard. There is a stump where the tree used to be and it is carved into a small chair. The base is about a foot high and there is a back support rising another foot and a half.

"What's this?"

"This is your special chair."

My eyes open wide. "Can I try it out?"

"Of course, it's yours!"

I slowly bring my butt down on the stump. I rest my back on the backrest. The chair fits my small body perfectly. This is one of the best surprises ever! I decide to forgive Dad for cutting the tree.

"How old was this tree, Dad?" I ask as I get up and wipe the dust from my butt.

"I'm not sure. Let's try to count the number of rings in the stump."

"Okay."

We kneel down next to the stump. I count, "One, two, three..." as Dad moves his index finger to each new ring.

"...sixty-eight, sixty-nine..."

We keep losing our place at seventy rings.

I decide to call it "the magic seat". It's in the coolest spot, right behind home plate in my backyard wiffle-ball field. All summer I invite kids to play in my new stadium and any time someone scores a run he gets to sit in the chair. I announce the players and pretend that the planes passing overhead are the planes that pass over Shea Stadium. I imagine the people by the windows in the airplane are pointing to us as they fly over, telling everyone else on the plane to look at the great baseball stadium below.

Late in the summer, Pat Hayes and I are about to start a phantom runner one-on-one wiffle-ball game when my father's car pulls in the driveway. I run over to greet him.

"Dad, we want you to throw out the first pitch! We're honoring the stadium builder today!"

"The stadium builder?"

He begins to laugh. I don't know why he is laughing. Soon he stops laughing.

He loosens his tie and walks toward the pitcher's mound. I scream out at the top of my lungs, "Ladies and gentlemen, if you would please direct your attention to the pitcher's mound!! Throwing out the first pitch is the builder of our stadium, Daaaaaaad Murphy!!"

Dad cocks his arm back but forgets to kick his leg in the air like a pitcher does. He has working man form, not pitcher's form and he throws high and a little wide. Pat makes a nice catch.

"Good luck guys!" Dad says as he goes inside to get changed and grab a cold beer, Genesee Cream Ale. In the first inning I look up to the deck. Dad has the Genny in one hand and his other arm around Mom and they are watching the game.

"The lovebirds are out tonight in this sellout crowd!" I scream.

• • •

We are at the man-made pond in Woodbury on a Saturday afternoon. I want to show Dad how well I can swim. I've been taking lessons.

I walk into the shallow end and he stands a few feet away from me.

"Swim to me, Kev!"

I start my swimming stroke just like they taught me, and when I get to where Dad should be he is still a few feet away.

"Keep coming, Kev!"

I swim a little farther but still don't reach him and I begin to suspect he is moving backwards each time so I take note of where he is standing and begin to swim again. When I stop, he is still a few feet away.

"Stop moving!"

"I'm not moving."

"Yes you are, you're moving backwards!"

"Well, you need the swimming practice. You have to swim more than just a few feet. Tell you what, if you can catch me I'll buy you an ice cream."

Mom is in the water now and sees me swimming and him backing up. She goes behind him and motions me to come. I start swimming. One Mississippi, two Mississippi three Mississippi, four Miss...Klunk! I get stopped by two big legs. They're attached to the man who has to buy me ice cream. He is dunking Mom.

• • •

We are having a really cold winter. We are not spending as much time playing outside 'cept to throw snowballs sometimes so we have started doing jigsaw puzzles in the house.

Danny, Patrick, and Dad set up the puzzle pieces on the dining room table each night and work on it for an hour or two. They're really hard puzzles and I can't help too much. I hate missing all the fun.

So Mom buys me my own puzzles, and when Dad and my brothers are finished for the night I spread my puzzle out on the table and ask Dad "Can you help me?" and he comes to sit at the table and I ask "Where do you think this piece goes?" and "How come this one doesn't fit?"

But I don't want too much help. I want him to watch me and see that I can do puzzles too. He sits there and watches, and is impressed by my skills.

"Where do you think this one should go, Kev?"

"Well, you see it's blue and has an end. It probably goes at the top as part of the sky."

"You're getting good. Soon you'll be able to do the big ones."

"I know."

• • •

Saturday afternoon. Dad is in the middle of working on something in the garage.

"Dad, can you sign this for me?"

He laughs as he shuts off the band saw. "Kev, the last thing you asked me to sign was a permission slip for a field trip and you wrote '911' as the number to call in case of emergency."

I don't know why he is laughing. Soon he stops laughing. He motions with his fingers. "Let me see what you've got."

"It's my cub scout book. I just need two more tasks in order to get my bear badge at the next meeting. Even Stanley Dickel has his bear badge. You can sign it now and we can do the tasks another time, when you're not so busy."

Sawdust falls from his hands as he says, "We can't do it that way" and grabs the book.

"Aaah, the infamous knots section. When is the meeting?"

"Monday. I don't know anything about knots."

"Why do you always wait for the last minute on these things, Kev?"

He looks through the pages in the book.

"Okay, I know a few things about knots. I'll tell you what. I'll find some time this weekend to work on it with you. Then I'll sign you off. Deal?"

"Deal."

After church on Sunday Dad teaches me about knots. The next day I impress Mom by tying my own shoes.

FIVE

Chemotherapy, Radiation, and Prayer

"Everybody take out the assignment and turn to page fifty-seven in the text book," my professor said as I sat in the back row in my Aviation History class on Tuesday. But my mind was on Dad. Was everything going okay? What was the chemotherapy like? The radiation? How was he reacting to it?

Mom and Dad arrived at Good Samaritan Hospital on October 18th like two people standing on a hill at the beginning of a sandstorm. Dad was quickly taken to the operating room to put the mediport in his upper chest, and a nurse directed Mom to the waiting room. She hated not being with him. She wanted to comfort him throughout; she wanted to hold his hand so that he felt her closeness during the procedures. But she wasn't allowed. She had to go to the waiting room and be alone with her thoughts while she hoped for the future and prayed for Dad. Meanwhile, Dad was alone with the doctors and all their tools, and he thought about Mom and hoped and prayed that she would be okay by herself.

The purpose of the mediport was to disperse the chemotherapy medicine into a number of different veins and throughout his body. The chemotherapy was designed primarily to stop the cancer from spreading to other parts of Dad's body. It was a continuous treatment for 96 hours, followed by a recovery period of three weeks before returning for a second cycle. Radiation treatments were scheduled five days a week during this same time period. Dad was warned about side effects from the chemo and radiation such as fatigue, vomiting and possible loss of hair.

Losing your hair while undergoing cancer treatments is very common, and I thought about how Dad would deal with it. If he lost his hair, I was planning to shave mine also, so that he would feel some solidarity between us. It was a silly thought, I know, but it was something I wanted to do for him.

The doctor administered anesthesia and Dad fell asleep for the mediport procedure. They opened an area underneath his collarbone and inserted the mediport beneath the skin. The procedure took about twenty minutes. When Dad woke up he was in mild pain. A little while after, they took him for his first radiation treatment.

What is radiation like? I thought to myself while we were going through our assignment in class. All I really knew about it was what I had read in the book, the book I took to the racquetball tournament. The book defined it as high-energy rays used to damage cancer cells and stop them from growing. But it didn't tell me if Dad was scared, if he felt alone, if he wanted to run out of the room and call the whole thing off. It didn't tell me who was in the room with him, what the technician said, if anyone would realize how special he was, if anyone would ask him if he was okay, if anyone would care what he was going through.

I prayed in my class as the professor began a discussion of U.S. Air mail. *God, please bless Dad and be with him.* I felt a burning inside my heart from wanting to know the future, the outcome.

A male tech brought Dad into the room where his radiation treatments started. They called the place where he laid a "treatment couch". It's a nice name for something so terrifying. The tech instructed Dad where to lie on the couch and walked out of the room and turned on the radiation beam. Dad felt no pain. No heat. No noise. Emphatically nothing. And that, I imagined, may have been scarier than any noise, heat, or pain he could have endured. It was just him and the radiation. Alone. The two of them, partners in this new battle. Dad began to pray, reciting the *Our Father*:

> *Our Father,*
> *Who art in heaven,*
> *hallowed be Thy name;*
> *Thy kingdom come,*
> *Thy will be done,*
> *on earth as it is in heaven.*
> *Give us this day*
> *our daily bread;*
> *and forgive us our trespasses,*
> *as we forgive those*
> *who trespass against us;*

and lead us not into temptation,
but deliver us from evil.
Amen.
Our Father,
Who art in heaven,
hallowed be Thy name;
Thy kingdom come,
Thy will be done,
on earth as it is in heaven.
Give us this day
our daily...

"It's over," Dad heard the technician's voice.

That was it. His first radiation treatment was finished. The tech helped him up. It was that quick.

They wheeled Dad up to his room on the third floor, where he would stay for the four days of chemotherapy treatment. He lay in the bed, a nurse came with a long needle, and Dad felt a sharp pain pierce through the soreness underneath his collarbone as she attached the needle to the mediport. Then the nurse checked the IV for the proper drip, and the chemo was under way.

In the waiting room, while all of this was going on, Mom was alone. She tried not to think about the radiation, the mediport operation, or the chemotherapy. She tried not to think about Dad being alone, she only wished she could have been with him. She thought of all the things they had done together, all they had been through. She hoped for their future, and she remembered their past, how meeting Dad had fulfilled her life.

Mom met Dad shortly after high school. She had become friends with a girl named Joan Kelley, who graduated with her from the Mary Louis Academy in January of 1957. She and Joan knew each other only slightly until discovering they were both going to work for the FBI after graduation. Dad had already been working at the FBI for several months.

After a month at the job, Joan told my mother about Dad. She described him as "a funny guy named John". One Friday, as they were sitting on the train about to leave the 59th Street Station, two hands peeled apart the closing doors and on stepped my father, a young man in a beige trench coat sporting a flat-top haircut. According to Mom, he was six-foot tall with a solid build and handsome.

"That's the guy I was telling you about! John Murphy!" Joan excitedly told Mom.

After that, Dad began seeing them more often on the train and after a few weeks he surprised my mother by asking her to the FBI dance. She had thought he was going to ask Joan.

It was raining the night of the dance, so Mom's parents, the Cronins, drove them so their clothes wouldn't get wet. Dad thought Mom was warm hearted, pretty, and had a nice smile, and as they sat in the back seat of the orange 1941 Ford, he took her by surprise, reaching over to put his hand on hers. Though Mom didn't know him very well at the time, she felt something tingle inside her at the touch of his palm and knew she was going to fall in love with him.

In the weeks following the dance, Mom and Dad sat next to each other on the train. Some days Dad got out a few minutes late, and on those days Mom waited for the next train. When he came down the stairs to catch the next train, she pretended not to notice him until he came over and said, "Hi Miriam. You still here?"

"Oh, hi. What a coincidence. You missed the first train too?" she would pretend.

As they began to enjoy each other's company more, they began using the slower "local" train so they would have more time to talk. Soon, Dad began taking Mom's bus with her after the train in order to see her all the way home. "I just want to make sure you make it home safe, with crime being the way it is and all," he told her.

Mom was dating someone else when they first met, but just before meeting Dad she had downgraded their relationship from "steadies" to "just dating." In the summer of 1957 she went out with Dad on Friday nights and Sunday afternoons. Saturday nights she went out with the other guy, Bob. It was a problem for Dad to see her on Sundays because the Cronins ate their big meal around 1:00 pm, while the Murphy's dinner was usually ready about 5:00. He couldn't pick her up until after 2:00 when she was finished with dinner and that didn't give him enough time to get home for his dinner after seeing her. His solution was to sacrifice dinner and eat peanut butter and jelly sandwiches.

Mom bought her own car soon after joining the FBI, but in the 1950s, the girls couldn't very well pick the guys up. It wasn't proper. It was a general rule that the guy courted the girl, not vice versa, and Mom and Dad followed this rule. When they had a date, Dad rode the bus to Richmond Hill and rang the bell to call for Mom. That was when the date started. After that, it was acceptable if she drove.

They went to see movies or to a drive-in diner for a hamburger, and sometimes they just drove around. They frequented a couple of nightclubs in Elmont, and went for strolls on the boardwalk during the summer along Rockaway Beach. The date would officially end when Mom drove them back to the Cronin residence. She couldn't drive Dad home because of the "courtship" rules, so Dad would say goodnight and run across the street to catch his first bus on the way home. Depending on the scheduling, it sometimes took him up to two hours to get home on the bus.

During the cold months of January and February of 1958, Grandma Cronin felt sorry for Dad having to stand outside waiting for a bus. A few times Grandpa Cronin agreed to drive with Mom to take Dad home because it was so cold. As long as he was in the car, the rules of courtship were intact. Around that same time, Mom went on her last date with Bob and became "steadies" with Dad. One day, Grandpa Cronin allowed my father to borrow Mom's car and bring it back the following morning. When Grandpa walked into the kitchen and handed Dad the keys, he was encouraging their continued courtship. It was as if he was handing Dad the keys to his only daughter. Dad vowed that he would never disappoint Grandpa Cronin.

Dad was nervous when, on an August night in 1959 he proposed to my mother. They had been dating for more than 2 years, had been "steadies" for over a year and they were in love. They had talked to each other about God and about what family meant to them. Mom remembers Dad as being fidgety all night. They walked along the boardwalk at Jones Beach and then along the sand. They looked at the ocean and the stars. Dad had prayed to God for weeks, asking Him to let Mom love him as much as he loved her. Mom had been thinking about the proposal for weeks and already knew her answer. Dad stopped near the water and looked back at the footprints in the sand. He reached for the ring in his back pocket and dropped to one knee. "Miriam, will you marry me?"

Mom began to cry. "Oh my gosh, yes!" she screamed.

As she sat in a chair in the waiting room, Mom recalled the proposal and seeing her mother's reaction when she told Grandma the news. "Break out the booze!" Grandma screamed. That was the beginning of their life together, a life filled with love and laughter and getting through some tough times in the early years of their marriage. But the proposal was another time and another place, and now Mom sat in the hospital waiting room, a room that would become the citadel of all her hopes and dreams for the future. What would the future hold? Would there be pain? Would there be suffering? Would there be any future at all for the two of them together? She thought about these uncertainties as the nurse came to fetch her and bring her to Dad's room.

Mom and the nurse took the elevator to the third floor, walked down the hall, past the nurses' station and made a right turn into the room. Dad was sitting up in bed.

"Miriam!" Dad yelled as he saw her enter the room. He motioned toward his roommate. "You know, hon, the food is so good here, he decided to go home *after* lunch."

Dad was in good spirits and was joking with his roommate. His roommate was a black gentleman from Orange County, a retired Army officer who had his face badly scarred during a bombing in the Vietnam War. He was a large person and in the hospital for high blood pressure, but was leaving later that day. Dad had been talking to the man and his wife before Mom came into the room.

Mom would have preferred that they could be alone for a little while, she wanted some private moments with Dad. She was worried sick. She didn't know how to take his comments. She wasn't in the mood for humor. She was overwhelmed with all the stuff he was hooked up to, the myriad of doctors and nurses involved, and this was only the beginning. But she didn't want Dad to know about her worries. It would only have worried him. So she tried her best to seem at ease.

"After lunch? Is that right?" she said. "And how about you? How are you feeling?" she asked as she reached his bedside and carefully hugged him, being sure not to put pressure on his sore chest or to disturb the IV or any of the other wires he was hooked up to.

"Yeah, I'm feeling pretty good, actually. It's not as bad as I thought. It's nice to finally see you again."

After only a few minutes together, a nurse came into the room and began to explain to Mom what all the hookups were for. "This is the IV for the chemotherapy, this is a vitamin supply to make sure he is getting all the nutrients he needs, this is to monitor his blood pressure and heartbeat, this is…"

Mom's mind blocked out the situation. She didn't want to know anymore. When the nurse finished talking, Mom told her, "I'll never remember all of those things."

"Don't worry," the nurse replied, "you'll know them all soon enough."

That statement hit my mother like a freight train on its way to Lake Erie.

It was yet another dose of reality, of what would lie ahead. It was a dose she didn't need at the moment. She felt her knees weaken, her eyes moisten, her heart race. She was halfway to hysteria and couldn't let Dad see her like that. He needed to keep his spirits high.

"I'll be back in a few minutes, John," she said in her calmest tone and walked out of the room. She barely reached the door when the tears began to pour. She walked down the hallway holding her hands over her eyes.

A plain-clothed woman, whom my mother would later discover was a Catholic nun named "Sister Sheila", passed Mom in the hallway and noticed her sobbing.

The woman reversed her direction and caught up to Mom and slowed to Mom's pace. "What's wrong, dear?" Sister Sheila asked.

"My husband is going through…" Mom couldn't even think of any of the technical names.

"…this and that and just had a mediport put in and he's hooked up to all these things and I *don't* know what they are and I'll never know and I don't care what they think I might get used to. I'll never get used to those things!" she screamed as she stamped her foot.

Sister Sheila put her hand on Mom's shoulder.

"And he has cancer!" Mom added.

The nun tried to calm Mom down as she spoke in a relaxing tone. "Who's the doctor?"

"Dr. Young," Mom told her.

"Well then, he's in good hands. I have a lot of faith in Dr. Young."

"You know him?" Mom asked.

"Yes, I do. But I'm more concerned about you right

now. Come, let's sit down over here," Sheila said as they reached a small waiting area and went inside to sit on the couch.

"So how are you holding up?"

"I'm a bit scared," Mom said.

"What are your fears, dear?"

"I'm scared about the cancer. I'm scared about what might happen. He's only fifty-five. I don't know what I would do if I lost him."

"Yes. I see God has thrown you a curve ball. You and your husband, you've been through tough times before, haven't you?" Sister Sheila asked as she put her hands over Mom's.

"Yes, we have," Mom told her.

"And how have you made out so far?"

"Pretty good, I guess."

"What makes you think this time will be any different?"

"I guess nothing."

"Well, there's something to think about."

The conversation was comforting to Mom, and she made a new friend. A little while later, the two women went to Dad's room where Sister Sheila was introduced to him. They hit it off right away, and when I meet Sister Sheila weeks later it seemed as if she'd known my parents since childhood.

•   •   •

I called Mom in the evening, after the treatments started. "How is everything?" I asked.

"Pretty good. The treatments went well. They started the chemo today and did the first treatment of radiation."

"Does he look okay?"

"He looks the same. Only he has the IVs hooked up to him. Other than that he's exactly the same."

"Did the doctors say anything else?" I was hoping for some new information, maybe a revelation about his condition.

"No," Mom told me. "It's just a slow process. They're not going to find out anything new right now. We just have to go through the procedures leading up to the surgery. All we can really do is pray."

I had been praying. I wanted to do more than pray. Wasn't there something more I could do? Just tell me how I can help, and I'll do it!

"You sound tired, Mom."

"I'm kind of drained. Emotionally drained. I met a nice woman today. She's a nun. She and Dad hit it off really well. She said she's going to visit with us every day."

"That's nice," I told Mom.

It was obvious that she was trying to keep a positive outlook on the situation. Whether it was for me or for Dad or for her I couldn't tell. I knew that inside she was worried, but it didn't seem the time to try to pry the worry out of her.

You see, cancer is a family disease; it never affects just one person. It alters the life and the outlook of an entire family, and often dominates their every thought, providing its own trials and tribulations. If things go well, cancer is normally a very slow process. It only speeds up when things go awry. Good news comes slowly, in drips and drabs, and is emotionally draining to the patient and their family. But bad news can come out of the blue at any time. And that is the test of one's nerves. If having cancer in the family was a job that you applied for, its main qualification would be patience. The patience it requires of the family affected is remarkable. It is as though we are helium balloons floating higher and higher into the air, needing to reach a certain height to be safe. We float slowly, higher and higher, and with each foot we become closer to our goal, yet the danger of popping becomes greater as we rise into the atmosphere.

The cancer family has only one goal: Health.

• • •

Dad was released on October 22nd.

"Don't be surprised if he starts vomiting a lot," one nurse told my mother.

"He'll be very tired," the doctor said.

One nurse confided some information to Mom. "He may not be the same person for a little while. He may be grouchy and easily irritated. Just give him some space if he needs it."

But chemotherapy and radiation has a different effect on each person, and can often affect them one way one time and a different way another. As for Dad, he felt surprisingly well after his four days in the hospital. Even his appetite had come back to him somewhat, possibly due to the shrinking of the tumor during radiation, and he asked Mom to stop for pizza.

I spoke to him that evening at the house. "I feel pretty strong, Kev," he told me. This was a small drip of good news, and it was welcomed.

God, thank you so much for looking out for my father, I started my prayer that night.

•   •   •

Dad convinced Mom that he could drive himself back and forth for the radiation treatments and that she should stay at the school district, as she was in charge of collecting school taxes.

While Dad went through radiation, I felt guilty at any enjoyment that I found in life. If I smiled at a pretty girl or laughed at a joke I would think to myself, "I shouldn't be enjoying this."

But life does continue, and that's one of the cruelties of cancer. As you wait for the next drip or drab of information, daily activities go on. I continued to go to school, I continued to work three nights a week at Aer Lingus, and I continued to have a beer a couple of nights a week.

•   •   •

I drove home to see Dad the weekend after he was released from the hospital. I approached the ninety-minute drive to Highland Mills much differently than the time I drove to see Dad after we had first found out he had cancer. I didn't think about what I was going to say this time, or about being careful. I didn't question whether it was okay to talk about the cancer. I simply put a Neil Young tape in my tape deck and sang along. Everything else would take care of itself when I got there.

Home was a relaxed atmosphere. Dad was happy to see me, and he showed me his progress on his carousel horse. He disappeared for a little while to work on the computer, and I watched Notre Dame play Navy.

After dinner I was sitting with him in the living room and felt the urge to tell him that I admired him. "I really admire the way you are going through this, Dad," I said as I sat on the piano bench watching the TV.

"What do you mean?" he asked from his chair.

"Well, you're so strong. In the head, I mean. I thought it would be hard to cope."

He gave me a modest smile. "Thanks, Kev, I really do appreciate it," he said. "There's not much I'm doing. These doctors are professionals. They know a lot more than I do about this stuff. So I just follow what they tell me to do."

"And the radiation, what's that all about?" I asked him.

"Well, it's designed to kill the cancerous cells without harming the healthy cells."

I wrinkled my nose and shook my head. I wanted to know more than that. "But what's it *really* like?" I asked him.

"Well, I lie down on a bed while some guy lines up the laser. Then they tell me there's nothing to worry about while they all run out of the room." He smiled sarcastically and motioned his fingers in a fast-paced walk across the arm of his chair.

"Then what?" I asked.

"Then I wait a couple seconds and this beam comes down on me. After a little while a man comes back into the room and tells me it's over. It doesn't take much effort on my part."

"Is it scary?"

He thought for a moment, then shrugged his shoulders. "A little bit," he told me in a soft voice.

"How long does it last?"

"One-and-a-half *Our Fathers*," he said.

SIX

Nine Years Old

We are at Aunt Jean and Uncle John's house near the ski resort at Hunter Mountain for a long weekend. There is a tennis court nearby and a couple of small ponds and a waterfall. On the ride up Dad tells me "I brought an extra fishing rod" and asks, "Would you like to try fishing with me?"

"Okay, I'll go with you," I tell him.

On the second day at the house we follow the dirt path and make a right turn just past the water tower and walk until we reach a small, deep pond.

It's been a few years since that first time I held a rod the day Mom couldn't reach the mortgage. Since this is our first official fishing trip together, Dad takes his time to explain the ins and outs of fishing and helps me to set up my rod.

When he's finished with my line he shows me how to cast. I try it but can't get the line to go very far. "Use more wrist!" he keeps telling me but the pond is deep even near the edges so we don't really need to get the line very far.

I keep forgetting that we are supposed to keep quiet so we don't scare the fish away. "They can hear us if we talk loud," he reminds me.

But I keep yelling, "Look at that one, Dad!" every time I see a fish jump above the water.

By lunchtime we haven't caught anything and we are hungry so we go back to the house to eat. I tell Mom about the jumping fish and that Dad is really good at casting his line.

"I hope to be as good as him someday," I tell her.

• • •

"Hey Sharr—oooon," Dad screams.

Sharon is doing a duet on stage at Washingtonville Junior High during the annual Joan Butler's Dance Studio recital. I am bored, as any guy would be. Why did Dad and I have to come? Tap dancing is for girls. We should be home watching sports on television. But since I'm only nine I have to listen when they say, "We're going here" or "We're going there". The only good part is we usually go for ice cream after the recitals.

"I think she's the best one in the whole show, hon! I swear to you!" Dad says as he applauds.

My mother nods in agreement. The flavor in my gum is almost finished.

"Aren't you proud of your sister, Kev?"

"Yeah, she's great Dad," I say in sarcasm.

I begin to think I'm missing something. Why is Dad so interested? And why did he set up the basement so that Sharon could teach a dance class for little girls? Now there are girls I go to school with taking dance lessons from my sister in the afternoons until their parents come home from work and pick them up. How annoying for me.

After the show Dad gives Sharon flowers. He smiles and looks at her just like he looked at me when I scored the winning *goal in my soccer game last week. Does he think this is as important as sports?*

• • •

I'M SORRY FOR HITTING FRANK ON THE HEAD WITH MY LUNCHBOX

I'M SORRY FOR HITTING FRANK ON THE HEAD WITH MY LUNCHBOX

I'M SORRY FOR HITTING FRANK ON THE HEAD WITH MY LUNCHBOX

Mrs. Goldstein has supplied enough chalk for me to write this over and over until the rest of the third grade comes back from lunch.

Frank is a sixth grade bully who picks on everyone on our bus and steals their cupcakes in the morning. Yesterday, I was bringing a picture home that I made for Mom and he tore it up. We got into a fight and I grabbed my Star Wars lunch box and hit him with it. Klunk! Since it was metal, it cut him and he started to bleed. His mother called mine in the afternoon.

I thought Dad wouldn't understand and would be upset at me without considering how it happened. But he took it pretty well. He told me, "I believe you have the right to defend yourself, just don't use it as an excuse for getting into a fight."

• • •

"Dad, Timmy Owens says my teacher this year is going to be mean."

"How does he know that?"

"Because she used to teach at Pine Tree School and his brother's best friend had her last year. Her name is Mrs. Levine

and Tim says all the kids call her Mean Levine. I don't want to go into her class. It's not fair."

"You just don't pay any attention to that nickname. Just because someone else thinks she's mean doesn't mean she really is."

A few months later, I realize that Mrs. Levine isn't mean at all. She becomes my favorite teacher.

• • •

Dad is walking in the door with packages under his arm. He calls Patrick and me into the kitchen and lays the bags on the table and tells us "Open them up, they're gifts".

Gifts? It's not Christmas, or near either of our birthdays.

The first things we see inside the packages are a couple of round coins that read "Tuit" on one side. Okay, Dad is trying to be clever again.

"What's this mean, Dad?" Pat asks.

"Well, you guys always tell me that you'll do certain things like mow the lawn when you get around to it. So now you both have a round tuit. You have no more excuses!"

Dad laughs.

Okay.

We look further into the bags. Lots of stuff for our tropical fish: a new filter system, gravel for the bottom of the tank, a model of a shipwreck for the fish to swim in and out of.

I can't figure out why he bought all this stuff for us today. There are even gifts for Sharon and Danny when they come home.

"Why all these gifts, Dad?" I ask.

"I got a little bonus from work, for a suggestion I made, and I wanted everyone to share in it."

"Was it the commercial, the IBM one with the Rubic's

cube on it?" I ask excitedly.

"No, not as big of an idea as that, I'm afraid. My idea won't make us rich, but it'll buy your mother and I a nice dinner tonight. I'll tell you more about it later."

When they get back from dinner Dad tells me about the computer gizmo that he suggested should get hooked up to another computer gizmo in order to make the office more efficient. All I can relate it to is that George Jetson is always giving ideas to Mr. Spacely to try and get promoted. I picture Dad's job as being similar to George's.

• • •

It's the summer after our fishing trip together at Hunter Mountain and Dad asks, "You wanna go fishing this weekend?"

"Fishing? Yeah, cool! Do you think we'll catch one this time?"

"Let's hope!" he says.

He leaves work early on Friday and we drive to a campground somewhere in Pennsylvania. We find a spot near the lake and pitch the tent. Saturday we get up early and begin fishing. By lunchtime Dad catches two fish but says they're too small and we have to throw them back even though I want to fry them up and eat them.

Mom made us sandwiches for the trip and we go back to the campsite to eat them on the picnic table and Dad and I talk.

"Do you think I'll ever catch one?" I ask him.

"Yes, I do. Just give it time."

In the afternoon we go back to the lake to fish and I feel a tug.

"Do you think I've got something?" I ask Dad.

He sees my fishing rod bending. "Pull the line in fast!" he screams.

As I struggle with the fish he gets the net ready and says, "Ease it in, we don't want to lose her."

I don't know how he knows it's a her but I don't ask.

I struggle with the fish, using all my muscles to reel her in. She's heavy! Must be a big one! Finally I get the line out of the water. Whew, what a fight!

"Ah, a nice little fish," Dad tells me.

"I don't see it!"

"Look at the end of the line," Dad says.

There is something small and shiny at the end of the line and I bring it toward me. As it gets close I can make it out. It's a tiny, measly, ugly, small, little fish!

"Is that it?" I ask.

"Either that's it or the rest of the fish will be here in a minute!" Dad says and begins to laugh and does that thing that Dads do when they put their hand on your head and mess up your hair.

I start laughing with him. The fish is at the end of the line. She's the only one that doesn't think it's funny.

He shrugs his shoulders. "Hey, it's a start, Kev."

"I guess. Can we keep it?"

"No. She's too small."

"Ooooooooooh!"

"You go stand by the fish so I can take your picture before we throw her back."

"You think anyone will see the fish?" I ask.

"Yeah, we'll make sure that they do."

SEVEN

Time is Torture

The image of Dad reciting the *Our Father* one-and-a-half times every time he went for radiation dominated my every thought for several days. That one sentence will stick with me for all eternity. He was spiritual, yet realistic. He wanted to live so badly, yet he trusted his fate to God.

Dad was feeling well as he neared the end of the radiation treatments. The treatments and medicines were relieving some of the pressure and discomfort on his esophagus and he was able to eat a little better. He even had the energy to attend the woodcarver's meetings and to help Mom get her office set up for tax season.

He had started to help Mom at the H&R Block office when he retired from IBM in 1990. Dad had been working for IBM since 1960 when, at the urging of the best man at his wedding, Dom Stavola, he left the FBI to take a chance with the little known company. His most lasting impression of the company took place after less than three months of employment. Mom and Dad were getting married and Dad requested to take his one-week vacation for a honeymoon, even though he did not qualify for vacation time yet. Not only did IBM grant his request, they threw in an extra week's paid vacation as a wedding present. Dad first worked in a position that today would be called a troubleshooter, then in the 1970s accepted a job as a programmer. In the late 1980s and early 1990s, IBM hit a slow period and encouraged early retirement for workers who had been there for a substantial period of time. Though he was only fifty years old, he had been working for them for 30 years, and after long talks with Mom, he decided to take the deal that was offered. He intended to find other work soon, but instead concentrated on his many hobbies and projects and enjoyed himself.

It was around the time of his retirement when computers became necessary for most businesses, and Dad took up the task of setting up a computer network for Mom's H&R Block offices. Eventually, maintaining and updating the system, along with taking on a number of other maintenance and payroll duties, became a full time job for Dad during tax season. The other employees in the office called him "John-of-all-trades".

Dad had encouraged Mom to start at H&R Block in the mid-1970s when few married women were working. Mom had taken a free class in tax preparation to try to save the family money on taxes, and H&R Block offered her a job after it was over. After a few years of working in a small Monroe office with only a handful of employees, the man who owned the Monroe office, along with two other offices, passed away, and none of his heirs wanted to run a business. Mom was in the right place at the right time, and came to own all three businesses at barely any cost, and a partial split of the first year's profits. She eventually took the

Monroe franchise that had previously done its business out of the corner of a wholesale distributor, and turned it into the most successful H&R Block in the area. At its peak, she employed over 35 people in the three offices.

• • •

Dad went back to Good Samaritan on November 15th for his second dose of chemotherapy. The surgery was already on the books for December 12th. This treatment didn't go as smoothly as the first.

"He's throwing up a lot," Mom told me on the phone.

"What do the doctors say about it, Mom?"

"They say we were just lucky the first time that he felt so good. This is to be expected."

Dad was released on the morning of November 19th, but this time he was in no mood for pizza. The only thing he put in his stomach were the anti-nausea pills the doctors gave him, and he had a hard time keeping even those in his stomach. "Just take me home," he told Mom when they left the hospital.

Dad slept a lot the first night. Whenever he wasn't sleeping, he threw up. The first night home he threw up a dozen times. He felt a stinging raw pain in his chest and stomach from the vomiting.

On Thursday, there was a small Thanksgiving gathering at the house. I had to work, and Danny and Dianne stayed on Long Island for dinner with her parents. Only Grandma Cronin, Patrick, Sharon, and Jamie and Benjamin were able to join Mom and Dad for the holiday.

I felt a bit guilty about working. But I was in no position to take off—I would probably be fired if I called in sick, and the hours and days of the job fit in perfectly with my lifestyle at the time. I should have insisted on the day off or called in sick and taken my chances, it was just a job. Instead, I missed out on sharing in Dad's last Thanksgiving turkey.

Because I didn't go, it left Grandma and Grandpa Murphy with no ride up from Long Island. They traditionally spent Thanksgiving Day with us.

I'll never forget the Thanksgiving after we got our first computer, when personal computers first became popular. Dad wanted to show his parents the amazing things that computers could do. After all, he had worked with them since he was in his early twenties, and they had never used one.

So after a lively game of Crazy Eights, where Grandma won $1.05 from the rest of us, Dad sat his parents down in front of the new PC to see if Grandma could beat the computer at the game.

Dad typed in Grandma's name and set up the game, and when Grandma and Grandpa sat down in front of the computer, "WELCOME JEAN!!" came across the monochrome screen in big green letters. Grandma nearly fell off her chair!

"How does it know me?" she screamed.

"I told it you were coming," Dad told her.

"How do I say thank you?"

"Just talk to it," Dad smirked.

"Thank you, computer," she said.

Underneath each card on the screen were numbers and in order to play the card, you had to hit the number that corresponded to the card you wanted to play. Both Grandma and Grandpa caught on quickly, not bad for two people who still thought that a telephone was for emergency use only. Then Grandma saw her first eight.

"WHAT SUIT, JEAN?" came across the screen. Grandma turned her head to Dad, who was standing behind her, and lowered her brow in a puzzling look.

"How do you change the suit, John?"

Dad looked at me and smiled. I could tell he had a trick up his sleeve, so I kept my mouth shut.

"Try to get as close to the computer as possible and tell it what suit you want," he said with a straight face.

Grandma leaned her chair forward and spoke to the computer. "Hearts!" she screamed. Nothing happened. She looked at Grandpa. He shrugged his shoulders. The two of them looked back at Dad.

"Try it a little louder," he told them.

"Hearts! Hearts! Heaaaaaaarts! Nothing is happening, John!"

"Maybe if you both try it at the same time," Dad suggested.

All they had to do was to type the first letter of the word, H for hearts. I knew it, and of course so did Dad, but he was having too much fun watching their reactions.

So as Dad and I stood behind them with our best poker faces, Grandma and Grandpa leaned their chairs forward and got real close to the computer and begin to yell "HEARTS! HEARTS!" in unison.

"It's not working, John!"

Grandma took it out on Grandpa, as if it were his fault. "C'mon Grandpa, you're not yelling loud enough! The computer can't hear you!"

"Maybe if we try holding hands," Grandpa suggested, desperate for a solution.

So they held hands and yelled "HEARTS!!" but there was still no change.

"Kevin, you get in here too and try it with us! Computers like young people. Get over here!"

So I went between them and held both their hands. "Hearts!" I yelled with them, to no avail. Grandma logically determined that the computer was cheating and didn't want her to change the suit to hearts.

"Okay, if it's gonna play that way, we'll try spades," she announced.

So the three of us held hands, got as close to the computer as possible and yelled "Spades! Spades! Spades!"

Finally Dad couldn't hold it in any longer. He began laughing hysterically.

"What are you laughing about, John? *You* come over here and tell it I want hearts!" Grandma yelled.

"I'm sorry, Mom. You really don't have to yell at the computer. You just have to hit the first letter of the suit you want on the keypad. Push H for hearts."

Grandma turned back to the computer quickly and pushed H and the screen read: "YOU HAVE CHANGED THE SUIT TO HEARTS, JEAN."

She looked at Grandpa and hit him playfully across the chest. "That's your son!" she yelled as we all laughed.

• • •

Shortly after the second chemotherapy, Dr. Young, the surgeon, explained the details of the surgical procedure.

Dr. Corning, the cardiologist, would be present the

entire time to monitor Dad's heart. Three incisions were to be made: one in Dad's neck, one down his back, and a third atop the scar of his heart surgery incision. This would allow the doctors the full range they needed to cut through the fatty tissue surrounding the organs. They would then proceed with the removal of the tumor and inspect the lung to determine its status. If the lung was infected, Young would remove the top lobe. A feeding tube would be inserted inside Dad's body so that he could be fed intravenously. The gallstones they found would also be removed before closing him up.

Dad joked with Young, "Will you let the gall stone removal ride along free of charge as part of a package deal?"

Staples would be used to close the incisions. The whole process was expected to take eight hours. After the surgery, Dad would be placed on a respirator. He'd stay in the recovery room until showing enough satisfactory progress to release him to the Intensive Care Unit. It would likely be twelve to eighteen hours before he woke up, and several days until he could breathe on his own. The staples would remain for six weeks.

The recovery, Young said, was going to be an arduous process *if* everything went well. Dad would be on a liquid diet, fed intravenously for at least a week, and wouldn't be able to walk for at least ten days after the operation. It would be several months before he could drive again. If all went well and he kept himself healthy, he would be eighty to ninety percent recovered from the operation in nine months to a year.

I had been a little concerned as to why they would wait so long between the radiation and surgery. Dianne became a nurse in 1993, and when I asked her about it, she had the same reaction.

"The doctors feel the tumor needs some time to shrink," Dad told me on the phone when I asked him. That seemed logical enough to me and Dad was confident in what the medical team was doing so I didn't ask any more questions. But the time in between was a detriment.

Dad stayed busy during the four weeks in between the chemotherapy and the surgery. After the vomiting days following the chemotherapy, he began to feel well. He did some woodcarving, read some books, and saw a couple of movies with Mom. He looked so good to me that it seemed nothing was wrong anymore. *Did the cancer go away? Are we out of danger? Is it all smooth sailing from here on out?*

The surgery, however, weighed heavy on Dad's mind. He was like a place kicker on a college football team whose opposition calls a time out just when he's ready to go out on the field and kick the winning field goal. The kicker usually tries to keep himself busy by getting a drink or readjusting his helmet. Like the kicker, Dad had plenty of time to think about what might happen.

As for me, I distanced myself from everything. It seemed so far away, and Dad seemed to be doing so well. Things had gone well thus far, and I didn't think anything could change. It was like a checklist:

> *Radiation—check*
> *Chemotherapy—check*
> *Surgery—on deck*
> *Recovery—standing by*
> *On with life—just down the road*

I retreated from the entire situation, repressing even the slightest of my fears. I went to school, played racquetball tournaments, drank beers, and chased girls. I saw Dad on some weekends, but refrained from any discussion about the cancer or the surgery. I couldn't deal with the time in between; the time to think about what might happen.

EIGHT

Eleven Years Old

We are watching the Cowboys vs. 49ers for the NFC championship. Patrick and I are rooting for the Cowboys, Danny and Dad for the 49ers. The Cowboys almost make an interception at the beginning of the second half and I get excited.

"Almost had it!" Dad says.

I turn to him in surprise. "Aren't you rooting for the 49ers, Dad?"

"I am."

"But that was the Cowboys."

"Oh, they changed sides?"

I nod my head.

"I forgot about that rule," he says. "You know, I understand why they change sides, but I think all the cameramen should change to the other side so the fans don't get confused."

Huh? Only Dad.

Late in the game, Dwight Clarke catches a fourth down pass from Joe Montana to win the game for the 49ers. As San Francisco celebrates the victory which sends them to the Super Bowl, I insist the television be shut off, and when nobody listens I run down the hall and slam my door.

Dad doesn't like it when people slam doors in the house. It's a "lack of respect" he says. Five minutes later he's sitting on my bed having a conversation with me.

"You have to learn to be a more gracious loser, Kev. You can't always win."

"I know."

"That's not all that's bothering you though, is it?"

"Well, no."

"What else is going on?"

"I don't know."

"C'mon, I'm your father. Tell me," he says as he throws his hands in the air.

"Well, we went to the store today and Danny wanted something and I wanted something. Danny got his because he has his own money. I don't have any money."

"Hmmm, I see. Maybe you should get an allowance if you help out around here. Are your friends getting an allowance?"

"Yeah, almost all of them. But I know we don't have so much money. Besides I don't like the word allowance."

He shakes his head. "Well, we don't have so much money, but we're not poor either." He puts his thumb up to his lips.

"I'll tell you what," he points at me excitedly. "Tomorrow I'll show you how to take in the garbage cans! And there are a few other things you can help out with too. Then we can call it…a 'salary' for helping out instead of an allowance. What do you think?"

"A salary? Sounds great! Do I get raises, too?" I say with a smile.

"We'll see as time goes on. How much do your friends get?"

"I don't know, I never really asked."

"How's a dollar-fifty a week sound?"

"*Pretty good, I can buy some good stuff with that!*"

"*Good. Then it's settled. Why don't you come back outside and sit with us? We won't talk about the game, okay? I promise.*"

"*Okay.*"

•   •   •

Dad and I are walking around the outside tables at the flea market in Maybrook. He is looking for anything interesting to use for a project. I am looking for baseball cards.

We come across a man selling various items. He looks like he emptied out his garage and put all the items on these tables. Dad picks up a few things but nothing interests him.

Wait a minute. Baseball cards! Stacks of them! Old ones! The sign says, "Baseball cards $1 per stack." I start to look through them. There are lots of cards from 1967-1973. Just the years I need. I count sixteen stacks and each one has about forty cards.

"*Look at these, Dad! Can we buy one?*"

"*Sure. Pick a good one,*" he says.

As I start looking through the stacks, we hear a voice coming from behind the table. "Please don't look through the cards, folks."

"*I just want to see which one to get, mister.*"

"*Well then just choose. I'm not letting people look through them. They're probably worth a lot more than I'm gonna get for them, I don't want someone picking and choosing. That's why I'm only charging $1 each.*"

Grouch. If you knew how much they were worth you would not be selling them, dummy.

"*Dad, how do I know which one to get if I can't look*

through them?"

"How much do you want for all of them?" Dad asks the man.

All of them, oh my gosh!

"I know I'm getting a bad deal on this one," the man says. "I'm sure they're worth a lot more. How's ten dollars?"

"Is that a good deal?" Dad asks me.

"Are you crazy? It's a great deal! Can you spend that much?"

"Well, let's see. I have eight dollars here." He turns to the man. "Can I bring you the other two dollars in a little while? I promise I'll bring it back to you."

The man agrees. We take all his cards. Dad finds Mom and gets two dollars from her to bring back to the man.

That night I have fun sorting through the cards and determining their value. They're worth well over a hundred dollars. Dad tells Mom, "He needs to learn a better poker face. I thought the man was going to take back his offer when he saw how excited Kevin was about getting them for ten dollars!"

• • •

Dad is playing with his hammer dulcimer; I am playing with my Superball. He likes the sweet tune the dulcimer plays; I like the bounce of the Superball. He is experimenting with various types of sticks to see which ones make the crispest sound. I am experimenting with different surfaces to see which ones make the ball bounce highest.

Soon our experiments cross paths. My ball rebounds off the wall toward the dulcimer, bounces off the strings and makes a twanging sound before rebounding into the dining room. Uh oh, I hope Dad doesn't get mad.

"*I like that sound!*" *Dad screams.* "*Hey, Kev, you have any more of those?*"

"*One more.*"

"*Do you think I could have this one?*"

"*For what?*"

"*I want to cut it up and attach it to the end of the sticks.*"

Attach it to the end of the sticks? A Superball? "*To play music?*" *I ask.*

"*That's right. I'll buy you a new one next time we're in town.*"

"*Well, okay.*"

So he chops up my Superball and shows me how to play the dulcimer with the new sticks. I bang the sticks on the chords. Twang! It does make a nice sound.

After a while I get my other Superball and start to play again. Dad spots me throwing the ball. "*Hey, that's got a different texture than the other one. Let's see how that one sounds!*" *he tells me.*

We bounce the Superball off the strings of the dulcimer. Sure enough, this Superball sounds a little deeper than the other one.

"*That's my last one, Dad,*" *I tell him.*

Soon we're in the car on the way to Shop Rite, loaded with quarters for the Superball vending machines.

• • •

It's near the end of summer and we are eating dinner on the back porch.

"*Are you excited about going back to school?*" *Dad asks.*

"*Not really.*"

I'll be happy to see my friends Jason and Kirk and a few

others, but I'm not excited about the schoolwork.

"What do you think your teachers will have you do when you start?"

I've already been around the block a few times and know the answer. "You know, the infamous 'What I Did Over Summer Vacation' essay."

"What are you going to write about?"

"I don't know. I'm going into seventh grade. I need a good story. Kids always read their essays about going to places like California, Disneyland, or even foreign countries. I never have anything exciting to write about."

"Why don't you tell them about the beach?" he suggests.

Jones Beach? That was fun. It was the first time I had ever been to the beach. Mom taught me how to ride the waves and Dad showed me how to swim under them. Mom told me that was where Dad had proposed to her. But it wasn't good enough for a summer vacation essay. "Too plain," I told Dad. "Some other kid probably went to Venice Beach."

"How about the Mets game we went to?"

"I'm sure somebody else went to three or four games."

"Well, you keep thinking about it," he says. "You're bound to come up with something."

The next day Dad tells me he has a couple of vacation days he could take from work and for me to try to think of something we could do, something I could write about in my essay. But I can't come up with any good ideas.

The following evening we are eating dinner on the picnic table on the deck and Dad says, "I was talking to Mom last night. I think I've got a good idea for your essay."

"Really?" I ask as I pour ketchup onto my french fries.

"I was thinking we could go to Cooperstown and see the

Baseball Hall of Fame."

I drop the ketchup bottle. "Are you serious? That's the best idea ever!"

Every boy I know starts dreaming about the Hall of Fame by the time he's eight. It's a place full of heroes. The place that is closest to paradise for boys. My friend Jeff's Dad says you have to go by the time you're fourteen or fifteen, or else it loses much of its magic, whatever that means. I've never been so excited!

We arrive in Cooperstown in the early evening on Wednesday. Dad takes a half-day at work, and it takes us four hours to get there from Highland Mills. We drive past "The Hall" and find a place to stay near the lake. When we wake Thursday morning, it's time to have fun.

"This is your trip Kev, you lead and we'll follow," Dad tells me.

So I walk, and Dad follows me with his camera, taking pictures that I will proudly take to school with me to prove my story.

There are trophy cases and uniforms for players like Cobb, Williams, Gehrig and Aaron. There are pictures and mementos of great World Series past. There are baseballs and reminders of events like Don Larsen's perfect game and Bill Mazeroski's home run; memorabilia from teams like the 1969 Mets and the 1954 Indians; feats like Roger Maris' 61 home runs and Joe DiMaggio's 54-game hitting streak. My parents watch as I get lost in the maze.

The second day we see a film on Babe Ruth and walk in the stands at the Hall of Fame ballpark. We go to a few of the shops and I buy some reprinted baseball cards of the 1927 and 1961 Yankees. We stop at a booth where you can test your arm against the speed gun—three throws for a dollar. I throw 49, 51, and 49 mph, and convince Dad to give it a try. 43, 38, 41. I win!

We finally leave The Hall at closing time Friday night. On the drive home I think about my essay and how I hope I can read it in front of the whole class.

NINE

Three Squeezes

In the weeks leading up to the surgery, I fell into a funk. There were no new developments; no drips, no drabs. There was just waiting. It was as if the entire situation became stale. Radiation and chemotherapy seemed years ago instead of weeks, and the fact that we were living with cancer began to seem normal. It was as if the cancer was gone, that it was a thing of the past. I put it out of my mind. Everything had gone pretty smoothly, and that was the only excuse I needed to deny all my fears. I repressed all bad thoughts.

I was at the house in Highland Mills eating breakfast Sunday morning, the day before the surgery. I had asked Mom and Dad their plan the night before and they told me they were going to mass at 11:00 and driving to the hospital after that.

"Want me to go with you, Dad?" I asked Sunday morning while picking up a glass of orange juice.

"No, it's not necessary," he told me. His voice was steady. "We're just going to fill out some papers and get checked into a room. You stay home and watch the football games. If you want, stop at the hospital on your way back to Long Island tonight."

So I stayed home and watched a preview of the Super Bowl as the 49ers beat the Chargers. At 6:30 I packed my stuff together for the trip back to Long Island and drove to Good Samaritan.

The walk to the room was sobering. This was a hospital, a real hospital. Dad was really here. He still had cancer. It hadn't gone away. We were still in danger. What had I been thinking these last few weeks? Where had I gone? Something in my head kicked me. It began kicking the walls of my skull. It was a monster or a witch. It began shouting at me to let it out. An image of Dorothy and Toto came to mind, "Toto, we're not in Kansas anymore," I heard Dorothy say.

I did my best to repress these images. Maybe they would go away, go to the place where all the other bad thoughts of the last few weeks had gone. Go away and don't come back. I don't want you!

When I reached the room, Dad was sitting up, staring down at a plastic table that straddled his body. On the table were a plastic cup, a pitcher of ice, and a gallon of what looked like water.

"What is that, Dad?" I asked as I entered the room.

"GAH-LEE-TEH-LEE," he told me. I looked at the side of the bottle. It read "Golytely". I assumed it was a play-on-words for "Go Lightly". But Dad insisted on referring to it as GAH-LEE-TEH-LEE, even though he knew that wasn't the correct pronunciation. I played along, because he seemed in the mood for a little humor.

It was beginning to hit me. This was it. It was real. The surgery was tomorrow.

Mom, who was in charge of the ice, was a little confused over the name on the bottle. She wasn't sure if we were kidding about its pronunciation.

"How does it taste, Dad?" I asked.

"It's horrible. I'm mixing it with half water. So it's like drinking two gallons of foul tasting water."

"Like Gatorade?" I asked him with a sideways smirk.

"I think it's even worse than Gatorade, Kev. Maybe more like warm Gatorade."

"Yuck."

After a few minutes a nurse came by and pointed at Mom and me. "I need you two guys to leave the room for a while. I have to do something with our patient here."

"Okay," Mom said. "Be back soon, hon."

"Yeah, don't go away, Dad," I joked with him.

So Mom and I walked down the hall until we found a waiting room. We sat next to each other on the couch. I smiled at Mom as I thought about what to say. She didn't seem to need the humorous statements that Dad wanted.

The monster in my head began kicking again. "Let me out!" he screamed. "I have all the bad thoughts and worries right here, now you let me out!"

This was bad. I'd just been ignoring the whole thing for the past few weeks, it seemed so far away. All of a sudden it was here and I didn't know what to do or say. It was like when we first discovered the tumor all over again.

Finally, Mom started the conversation. "How am I going to get the news to you after the operation?"

Mom's question landed like a hard slap across the face, and the monster inside my head broke another chain. I hadn't even made a plan for what I was going to do during the surgery, whether I would be at the hospital or stay on Long Island and wait for news.

I set myself up for the knockout blow. "Mom, how do you think this compares to the surgery he had a few years ago, the one on his heart?"

Mom seemed a little puzzled, as if she couldn't figure out why I would ask that sort of a question now. She narrowed her eyes and lowered her eyebrows.

I wanted her assurance that it wasn't so serious; I wanted her to tell me that I didn't need to worry. I wanted to ease my mind from the scary thoughts it was trying to hold back, I wanted to lock the monster up and never let him out.

"This is much more serious, Kev," she told me. That was the jab. The knockout blow came next.

"You know, Dad's very concerned about you, Kevin. He told me he didn't know how you were handling this whole thing. He knows how highly you think of him."

Had I been that bad that Dad had to be concerned with me instead of with himself? Had I made that mistake once again, only caring about myself and forgetting about him? I suddenly started to realize the stage to which my denial had escalated. Bang! The monster with all the fears was released.

Somehow, I was planning to go to school as normal the next day. After classes I would play racquetball, do some homework and go for a beer. At some point someone would call me and let me know everything was okay. What was I thinking?

I wanted to dig a hole right there and disappear. This denial of mine, was it obvious to Mom? Was it obvious to Dad? Did they think that I didn't care?

"Oh, Mom. Oh my God, Mom. What am I doing? What am I asking you?"

She didn't really comprehend what I meant, but as tears filled my eyes and poured down my cheek, she grabbed hold of me and we hugged on the couch.

I came to the realization of what was going on. It was like I was waking up. The monster was released, and now my fears poured out. It scared me, but it was a relief. That little guy was torture for those weeks. He had hid the truth. Now I could deal with him.

So what would I do? Why wouldn't I come to the hospital during the operation? I don't care about school. What am I going to miss? A class? Even if it were the most important class in my life, how could it compare to being here for Dad?

But I knew my parents. For me to miss school was for me to make them worry. They had enough worry.

"What time will the surgery be over, Mom?"

"It should be over around six o'clock."

"How about I come back tomorrow?"

"What about school?" she asked.

"Come on, school?" I looked at her with are-you-serious eyes. "I finish at two o'clock on Mondays. I can drive up right after that."

"Don't you have finals next week? Don't you need to study?"

School wasn't important anymore. Imagine something went wrong. I should be studying airline deregulation while my father is suffering, taking his last breath? No, I wouldn't let that happen. I should be with him. He will have a better chance to get through it if I'm with him.

"I can't concentrate on doing any schoolwork, Mom. I can leave after my last class and get here around 3:30. Don't say no, I want to be here."

She nodded her head. "Okay. Let's not tell Dad, though. I don't want him to be concerned about you with school."

"Okay, Mom."

Dad was concerned with how I was taking this. He knew I was denying it these last few weeks. Yet he let me, I guess he thought it was what I needed to do. He knew how much I thought of him and he expressed it to Mom. That was special.

Dad walked into the room as Mom and I were holding hands, and we both had moist eyes. He came over and put his arms around both of us and gave us a big hug.

"It'll be all right. Everything will be okay. Come on, no more of this crying stuff," he told us.

The three of us walked back to the hospital room together and talked for a while longer. We left the hugging and the tears in the waiting room. Mom and I didn't mention to Dad that I was coming back the next day.

I don't recall the particulars of what we talked about over that last half hour, but I do remember we told jokes and laughed quite a bit. I left at closing time, 8:30, but Mom convinced one of the nurses to let her stay past visiting hours. When I left, Dad still had almost a half-gallon of Golytely left. I walked over to the bed and kissed him. "Good luck tomorrow," I said. "You're going to do fine."

On the drive home I thought about what Mom had said to me, that Dad knew how highly I thought of him. This was something intimate Dad had shared with Mom, and I felt privileged that Mom shared it with me. I had often wondered over the last several years if Dad realized that I had grown to like him so much. It was nice to know that he *did* know and that he expressed this to Mom.

When I got home that night I prayed. *This is it, God. This is the big test. I know you'll be with Dad. Please be with me too, so that I can do whatever I need to comfort Mom tomorrow.*

•   •   •

At ten o'clock I was sitting in a Physics class and I imagined my father lying on an operating table as the doctors began to make the incisions. How many *Our Fathers* had he said this morning?

The Physics teacher talked about arms and moments and things of that nature. Who really cares? That stuff isn't important. The important stuff today is Dad.

The class crept along much like the cancer itself. I kept watching the clock. I didn't know why I was there. I guess it was so that Mom and Dad wouldn't worry about me *not* being there. I watched the minutes go by. At two o'clock, I packed my books, headed to the car, and drove to Suffern. Most of the ride I played the radio loud and sang along to the songs. I hit no traffic and arrived at 3:15.

I entered the hospital and sat on the couch in the lobby. I prepared myself for seeing Mom. What if she wasn't there? That would mean bad news. She'll be there. But what do I say? Oh, no, not this again. What *do* I say? Think, Kevin, think. Relax. Take a few deep breaths. Okay. Just say what comes to mind. No regrets. You'll know what to say. Say what you think you should. Comfort Mom, that's your job. Okay, time to go.

I walked down two long corridors toward the waiting room. One hundred fifteen steps. At the end of the steps I turned left into the doorway. I didn't think about what to say.

"There he is," I heard a woman say from the far right corner of the room. It was Mrs. McIntosh, a friend of my mother's. Next to her was another friend, Mrs. Reilly, and seated across from them was Sharon. I knew my sister had taken off from work and was going to be there the whole day, but I hadn't expected to see the others.

As I walked towards Mom I asked, "What's happening? Any news?"

"Not too much news. We're just waiting," Mom told me. I guessed that was good news.

When I reached Mom I gave her a warm hug, like the one Dad gave me at the top of the stairs when I first saw him after learning about the cancer. I squeezed Mom long and hard. I didn't want to let her go.

"How was the trip?" she asked as I let go of her body and took a seat across from her.

"Fine. No traffic. How was Dad this morning?"

"I was with him when they took him into surgery. They asked me to leave at a quarter to nine."

"That was the last time you saw him?"

"No, a half hour later a nurse came into the waiting room and asked me to follow her. She scared the life out of me! I thought something was wrong."

"Where did she take you?"

"I followed her to the surgical holding area, where Dad was lying in a bed still waiting to go in. She thought I might want to spend a little more time with him. They asked me to leave at 9:45. So they must have started around ten."

"Has there been any contact with the doctors since then?"

"No, we probably won't see them until six o'clock," Mom said.

As the five of us sat in the corner of the room, we found other things to do instead of talking about the surgery and the cancer. That would have been too stressful. There were hours of waiting left.

Mrs. McIntosh opened a large bag of Hershey's Miniatures and we all munched on those as we talked. I liked the Krackel candies the best, while Mom ate the Special Darks. There was a television high up in the opposite corner of the room tuned to the afternoon talk shows, which continuously brought us up to date on other people's personal lives. I was amazed at how many things I found out that really weren't any of my business. We talked about the television shows, and about food and about Christmas gifts.

After a little while, Mrs. Reilly started a conversation about Dad when she reminded us that her late husband and Dad were good friends. She said that Mr. Reilly was continually amazed at the conglomeration of items that Dad used to decorate the downstairs family room in our house.

"It was the 1970s. We had no money," Mom said. "We sacrificed ourselves to buy the house. So we improvised for the downstairs. We wanted it to be a place where the kids could hang out and bring their friends."

Dad started his decorations when my grandparent's church was cleaning out their basement and had some old instruments they were getting rid of. Dad claimed an accor-

dion, cello, bass drum, and a snare drum and put them in
the room along with an old couch that a neighbor was
throwing away. He also picked up three small decoration-
only type jukeboxes, a piano, and a big sign reading
"Murphy's Harmonica" which added flavor to the room. At
a garage sale one day he found a bumper pool table that was
inexpensive and that he thought would be entertaining. He
learned how to play and gave all of us lessons on the game,
and he and Mom decorated the walls in red and gold drap-
ery to match the red cement floor. The final piece to the
"entertainment center" was a jukebox.

"Remind me what happened with the jukebox, Mom.
Didn't we bring it to Long Island and then bring it back
again?" Sharon asked.

Mom snickered. It was nice to see her thinking about
a happier time.

"Mr. Ponikvar owned a jukebox from one of his stores
and wanted to sell it, but it was broken," Mom said. "They
asked Dad to pick it up and see if he could fix the problem
and bring it to the Ponikvar's home on Long Island."

She proceeded to tell the story of Dad driving to Chester
to pick up the jukebox, offloading it at the house and fix-
ing it. Then Danny and Patrick—I was only four years old—
helped Dad load it into the van and we all drove to Long
Island for dinner with the Ponikvars. Before dinner, they
offloaded the jukebox and brought it into the Ponikvars'
house, and during dinner my parents told the Ponikvars
that they wanted to buy it. Though Mom and Dad didn't
have the money, Mr. Ponikvar agreed to wait until their tax
refund came through.

"So we loaded the jukebox back into the van, again,"

Mom explained. "And we brought it back with us to Highland Mills, again."

"One play for a dime, three plays for a quarter," I said to my sister, reminding her of the sign on the jukebox.

"That was a great set-up you guys made for us," Sharon told Mom.

"Well, we wanted you guys to be comfortable hanging out at home instead of somewhere else," Mom told her. "We didn't have much money, but we did the best we could."

"Remember Richie Fabian on New Year's Eve?" Sharon asked.

"Oh yeah. That was funny," Mom remembered.

One particular New Year's Eve at the stroke of midnight, my godfather, Richie Fabian, grabbed the big bass drum and started banging on it. Then he opened the door and walked out to the street and proceeded down the block. Dad picked up the accordion and followed him, while Mom, Aunt Ida, and the rest of us kids grabbed pots and pans and spoons and anything else that would make noise and followed them down the street. It quickly became a New Year's tradition, and eventually many of the neighbors joined in too.

"You remember Johnny Whoops, Mom?" Sharon asked with a chuckle.

Johnny Whoops happened before I was born, but I knew the story well. My brothers and sister brought home a silly game from school. In the game they said the word "Johnny" when they touched the tips of each of their five fingers and "whoops" in between the index finger and the thumb. They then reversed direction and did it again.

Starting with the pinkie it sounded, "Johnny, Johnny, Johnny, Johnny, whoops, Johnny, whoops, Johnny, Johnny, Johnny, Johnny." At the end of the passage the person, or people, folded their arms together. The folding of the arms was the whole key to it. The rest was easy.

They tried the game on Dad but he did not fold his arms at the end. It lasted for over an hour, with each of the kids showing Dad how to do it. He promised them that if he could not figure it out by the time the ice cream truck came, they would all get ice cream as a treat.

"All of us did it together," Sharon said, "and even folded our arms as obvious as possible at the end."

"But John couldn't figure it out," Mom told her friends.

By the time the ice cream man came, Dad was still baffled and he had to buy everyone ice cream. They made the same bet the next day, and Dad wound up buying ice cream again.

"We asked if he wanted us to tell him the secret," Sharon said, "but he told us he would figure it out eventually!"

"He even got it right a couple of times by accident," Mom told the ladies, "but on his next try he didn't fold the arms. Before we went to sleep each night, he'd ask me if he was really missing something."

Finally, after three nights of ice cream, Dad suddenly erupted in laughter. He had figured it out! That story has lived on for decades.

"And Johnny McEldoo," Sharon said.

"Oh yeah," Mom said, "an Irish song from the Clancy brothers that John loved. He printed out the words and made all the kids memorize it. The song went faster and faster as it went on."

"Still, I think his best is the hole in the wall for the trains," Mrs. Reilly mentioned, referring to Dad's LGB trains. He made a tunnel for the trains to get from the living room to the dining room one Christmas by cutting a hole in the wall.

I started telling the story of his mailbox adventures. Dad had made a nice mailbox out of wood, and it was the best looking mailbox on the street. On each side, in large letters, he carved the family name and painted it gold, and next to the name he carved a little shamrock and painted it green. But it was knocked down by the snowplow. Dad was upset that the mailbox was knocked over by the plow, so he came up with a mailbox that couldn't be knocked over. He was always saving scraps and pieces that he thought might be of use one day, and he had some type of a bendable stick in the garage that he had saved. He connected the stick to a spring, and put a lightweight box on top of the stick. That way, if the plow or heavy snow hit the box, it will give a little, and then spring back to its original position when the force was removed.

"Leave it to Dad," I said, "there's always a way."

I remembered the next summer, it was a thrill for the kids in the neighborhood to ride past our house and bend our mailbox, so they could watch it spring back into place. The post could actually bend until the mailbox touched the ground!

Just as we were laughing about the mailbox, we heard the five o'clock news come on the television. That meant the end of the talk shows, and the beginning of the more serious news hour. It was also the end of our lighthearted conversations, as we figured we'd hear news about Dad within the hour.

The tension in the room increased. Mom's arms and legs bounced nervously and her eyes became moist. Her body flinched at various times. We fed her lines like "no news is good news" and "the doctors know what they're doing" and "everything will turn out all right". I went over to her and put my arms around her and gave her hugs. There wasn't much else we could do.

We were all hungry, so at 5:30 Sharon and I went to the cafeteria. I picked up a bag of Wise potato chips and a Snapple lemon iced tea. My sister grabbed a cup of tea and a snack for herself, and a muffin and black coffee for Mom. Sharon treated. On the way back to the waiting room we stopped to look at the clothes a charity organization was selling.

At six o'clock, I looked at Mom and her eyes were moist. Her legs were bouncing. She was grasping the fabric on her pants and pulling at it. I gave her another hug.

"You know, they may not have started at ten o'clock," Mrs. McIntosh reminded Mom in her calmest voice.

"The doctors were ready to start when I left," Mom insisted.

"Yeah, but you're not a doctor, Mom," I told her. "You don't know, maybe they had a lot of doctor things to do before they could start, and just asked you to leave so that they could go about doing them."

Mom appreciated our efforts, but our words didn't give her the comfort she needed. She wouldn't be satisfied until she saw her husband alive.

Mrs. Reilly called the hospital from the waiting room phone to see if she could get some information.

"Hi, I'm calling about John Murphy. He had surgery today," she said.

"Yes, I'm a relative," she lied to the woman on the other end of the phone.

"He is?" She covered the phone and looked to us excitedly. "She's pretty sure he's in the recovery room," she whispered to us. "She's going to see if she can confirm it."

We let out a collective gasp. For long seconds we hung on to the hope that he was in recovery and the doctors had neglected to inform us.

"Why wouldn't they have told us?" Sharon asked.

"Yes," Mrs. Reilly spoke again. "He's still in surgery? And there's no other news? Nothing else you can tell me? Okay. Thank you for trying."

There was no news.

As eight o'clock approached there was no more talk. We sat silent. We were the only ones in the waiting room. There had been others earlier in the day, but they were all gone. Every ten minutes Mom and Sharon got up and walked around the room and looked outside in the hall, hoping they would see a doctor approaching.

My optimism began to weaken for the first time. Will we ever hear some news? Or will Dad and the surgeons stay in the operating room forever and we'll never know?

Go to the chapel to pray, I heard a voice from inside of me.

"Do you want to go to the chapel with me?" I asked Mom.

"I was there earlier," she said. "I'm not leaving this room. This is where the doctors know they can find me."

"Okay."

"It might be a good idea if you go, though," she said. "Say prayers for the two of us."

So I went to speak with God.

The chapel was empty, just as I had hoped. I knelt down in front of the altar and prayed. First the *Our Father*, then *Hail Mary*, then my own. *God, please let my father be okay. We have so much left to do together. He has so much left to do on his own. Please let him be okay. I'll give anything. Take me if you have to take someone. He is such a good person, so good to others. He is so important to Mom and to the family. Please let him come through. I haven't been able to show him the love that he has shown me yet. He hasn't finished the things he wants to do. He's fighting hard. Help him to fight. Please dear Lord. Please.*

I hoped that upon my return from the chapel, my mother would have a smile on her face. But when I returned, she was still grasping at the fabric on her pants. There was still no news.

I was standing in the opposite corner from everyone else at 8:23 when a man in a doctor's getup walked into the waiting room. My mother had sat down only a minute before, but she erected herself in her chair the instant she saw him, so I knew this was the surgeon. I saw him squint his eyes as he tried to adjust to the light in the room. He looked into the corner and when he picked Mom out of the small crowd, he began to speak.

"The surgery went fine, Mrs. Murphy. He's in the recovery room now."

I pumped my fist into the air! I twirled my body around like an ice dancer in the Olympics and pumped my fist again! That was the million-dollar news! Sharon reached over and put her hands on Mom's. Mom let out a deep gasp and allowed her head to fall backwards. She was relieved, but didn't let herself lose focus on the doctor as he continued to speak. She nodded her head as he talked, but I caught only bits and pieces of what the doctor said. I was too excited! It was the most exhilarating moment I had ever experienced!

The doctor mentioned that the length of the surgery had to do with the tumor being larger than they had antici-pated. The gallstones were not removed because of the duration of the surgery, out of concern for his heart, but the good news was that a section of the lung had been tested and it was not infected with cancer!

As the doctor was leaving I shook his hand. He didn't know who I was, but it didn't matter. I went over to Mom and gave her another hug, the nicest one of the day.

I ran down the hall to call Grandma and Grandpa Murphy, while Sharon called Dianne, who in turn let Danny, Patrick, and Grandma Cronin know the good news. They, in turn, would relay the news to the Littmanns, the Pulvers, and the other friends who were waiting. There was a whole chain worked out.

Grandma Murphy picked up the phone on the first ring.

"Grandma, it's Kevin! Good news! Everything went fine! He's out of surgery and in the recovery room!"

"Have you seen him yet?" she asked.

"No, not yet, maybe a little later. But the doctor says he's okay."

We had a hard time convincing Mom that what the doc-tor said was nothing but good news, but she couldn't feel completely comfortable until she saw Dad. So, after going to Friendly's for dinner, Mom, Sharon, and I sneaked back into the hospital after visiting hours at 10:30.

We waited near the recovery room for half an hour, then saw Dad roll past us in a bed, accompanied by five hospital staff. We went upstairs to the intensive care unit, where a nurse was understanding of our situation and told us to let them get him settled in and then we could see him. She came back after fifteen minutes to get us.

"He won't be able to talk, but he can hear you just fine," the nurse told us as we were briskly making our way toward the room.

I looked at Mom in amazement over what the nurse had said. She lowered her brow in a confused look.

"You mean, he's conscious?" I asked the nurse.

"Yes he is," she said.

When we reached the room, Mom spoke to him first. She knew exactly what to say. I stood a few feet away, admiring her composure. She was like a priest before her congregation on a Sunday morning. She did a great job in calming Dad's nerves.

"Hey, John. You made it. The doctor said you're fine. It's eleven o'clock and we're just getting to see you for the first time." His eyebrows rose when she mentioned the time. "They looked at the lung, there's no cancer there. They said you're in fine shape."

As Mom held his hand, he responded to questions by squeezes in a code designed by the two six years earlier, just before his heart operation. One squeeze meant yes, two meant no, and three meant "I love you".

"Can you see Sharon?"

One squeeze.

"And Kevin?"

Two squeezes.

"Move closer, Kev," Mom ordered me.

I moved closer. "Hi, Dad," I said.

He gave me a brow raise. That was the only sign he could give me. I took it to mean he was happy I was there.

I was nervous when I finally got my chance to hold his hand. He seemed larger-than-life to me, and I was once again not sure what to say. With all he'd been through, I wanted to say something special. But words escaped me.

"You look beautiful," I told him. "I never saw you look so good."

Then he squeezed my hand three times.

The hardest part was over. He was going to be okay.

TEN

Changing Attitudes

Wednesday afternoon lunch recess. I am flipping baseball cards with a few of the guys at school and we are talking about our bedtimes and how we can extend them if there is a good show on television or something.

"Every Monday during football season my Dad lets me stay up and watch the first half of the football game," I tell them. I explain, "He says he's going to bed before me and gives me a kiss and says 'make sure to go to bed right after the first half is over'."

They laugh at me and one of them says, "Anyone who still kisses his Dad is gay!"

"Oh yeah, well I'm not gay," I tell them. "I really just made it up."

That night at bedtime I say "Good night Mom" and give her a kiss.

I walk over to Dad and say "Good night Dad" and hold out my hand. He pauses for a moment and gives me a puzzled look. I wonder what he will do. I don't want everyone at school to laugh at me because I kiss my Dad before bed. He looks to Mom and then back to me.

He takes my hand in his and squeezes hard. "Good night, Kev."

•   •   •

"I see you have your glove, want to have a catch, Kev?" Dad asks.

"No, it's okay. I'm going to play by myself and throw the ball against the wall."

I'm a teenager now and getting too old to have catches with Dad. It's not cool anymore. Everybody knows that.

"How about we shoot baskets, then?"

"No, not today. Maybe another time, Dad."

"Okay," he says as I pass by him in the garage with my ball and glove.

"Hey, Kev," he adds, "do you want to go fishing at one of the lakes this weekend?"

"Umm. I'll think about it, Dad. I'm not sure."

"Okay, you let me know."

•   •   •

6:30 pm. I am finished eating dinner and get up from the table.

"Hey, where you going?" Dad asks.

"To play a little bit."

"Sit down for a minute. Why don't you tell me how school was today?"

I sit back in my chair. "It was okay."

"What did you do?"

"Nothin'."

"Didn't you learn anything today?"

"Mmmmmmm, not really."

"Okay. So what are you going to play?"

Dad has this habit of asking me to share things with him. Why can't he leave me alone sometimes? Doesn't he realize I'm a teenager and I don't need this anymore?

"Probably play Atari, or flip baseball cards."

"Baseball cards? Get any new ones?"

"Of course, I get new ones every day at school."

He smiles. "Maybe that's why you're not learning anything."

Is this going anywhere? Can I go now?

"Well, I can see you have things to do so I won't keep you," he says. *"Can you ask to be excused from the table?"*

Uh oh. I hate the words 'may I be excused'. Like adults have bad words, usually the four-letter kind that Mom and Dad don't let me say in the house, kids have their own bad words. 'May I be excused' is at the top of the list for me. It's the first time in a long time that I have been asked to say them. Last time I almost threw up afterwards.

I notice Patrick is finished eating now too. He gets up without a word. Now is my chance to get out of this.

"Nobody else has to say it!" I tell Dad.

Pat runs back to the table. "May I please be excused?" he says with a smirk.

"Yes, you may," Dad tells him.

PATRICK!!!! I hate you!! I'm going to kill you!

"Well, I don't want to say it!" I tell Dad.

"Then I guess you really don't want to play, do you?"

"Mom, why do I have to say it?"

"Because it's polite. They're just words, Kevin, it's not a big deal," she says.

"Well I don't like those words. I'm not going to say them."

"Suit yourself," Dad says. "But you're not leaving the table until you say them."

Dad grabs the newspaper and starts to read. Mom looks at me, obviously disapproving of my stand.

I wait.

Seven o'clock. Seven-thirty. Dad gets up from the table. "I'm going to the living room. If you want to be excused just let me know and I'll come back in."

I don't say a word.

Eight o'clock. Eight-thirty. They wouldn't make me sleep here. Surely they'll give in soon.

Nine o'clock. Dad comes back into the kitchen. "So do you have anything you want to say?"

I shake my head.

"Well, dammit! Just go to bed then!"

"Dad? Don't get so upset."

Mom runs into the room.

"For three hours he can't say four simple words! I can't take it!" he tells her.

"May I be excused, Dad?" I scream from my chair.

"It's too late! You've already been excused!" He storms out of the room.

"Mom, why is he so upset?"

"Because of the way you acted. First you can't even talk to him a little and tell him how school is going. And then you disrespect him. He gives you three hours to make good on it and you can't even do that. Just go to bed!"

I walk to my room, head down. I feel bad. I still don't like those words. Next time I'll say them, though, even if I do have to throw up afterwards.

ELEVEN

Red Sweatpants

The day after the surgery, I breezed through my classes. The teachers were getting us ready for finals and all I could do was smile. They had no idea what my soul had been through the day before. It was like I won the lottery. I thought about Dad all day, and when the classes were over I drove back to the hospital to see him.

Danny was in the room when I got there at five o'clock. He had left work early to visit with Dad. I barely missed seeing Mom. She was there all day but left five minutes before I arrived to attend a meeting.

"Hey, Kevin," Danny said with a surprised look as I entered the hospital room. I hadn't told anyone I was coming.

"Hi, Dan," I said as I walked in and gave him a hug.

Dad spotted me right away, and to my astonishment, he was able to talk. "Kevin, what are *you* doing here?"

He was off the respirator already, although he was hooked up to oxygen and another machine that covered his mouth and made his voice different. He sounded like Darth Vader from *Star Wars*, but I was happy just to hear him talk.

"Well, I really needed a break from studying and decided

to take a ride," I told him as I approached his bed and put my hand on his. "There was no traffic on the road and I just wanted to come and see you."

He nodded his head slowly. He looked like he wanted to smile but it was too difficult for him.

"Well, I'm...glad you're here," he told me.

That alone made it worth the trip.

There was a sponge next to his bed that Danny used a couple of times to wet Dad's mouth. He wasn't allowed to drink any liquids yet, so his mouth was very dry.

"What are these things?" I asked Dad as I pointed to the liquid bags on the pole.

Danny answered for him. "This one is his food and the other one is a painkiller," he explained.

"It's pretty neat," Dad interjected with his Darth-Vader-like voice. "If I have any pain I just hit the button and it gives me a dose. It's governed to keep me from overdosing."

"Wow, cool," I told him.

It was such a great feeling I had. I couldn't stop smiling. I was the lottery winner, on cloud nine. With all I had taken for granted in my life, with all I had missed, I now had the chance to make up for it. Dad, who I failed to appreciate for all these years, was going to be okay. I pictured going to the Gettysburg museum with him as we had talked about; I pictured him filling up the new photo albums he had recently bought; I pictured him and Mom going on trips together; I envisioned us going fishing together again.

I was there only a few minutes when Dad began falling asleep. He had been through so much. He was tired. It wouldn't be right to make him stay awake to talk to us.

"Dad, I think you should get some rest," Danny told him.

"Mm-hmm," Dad mumbled as he closed his eyes.

"We'll go," Danny said.

"Okay. I'm sorry guys," Dad told us as he fought to open his eyes again. "I just don't think I can stay awake."

It was fine with me. Just those few minutes there were quite fulfilling.

"Okay, Dad. See you in a few days then," I said as I gave him a kiss.

"Thanks for coming," he said to me.

Danny and I went across the street to get a bite to eat at the diner. We talked about Dad. Danny asked what my day was like in the waiting room. He told me of the nervousness he felt all day waiting for news about the surgery. We talked about Dad and about the recovery phase. As we sat eating hamburgers, we were both confident of Dad's recovery.

• • •

On Wednesday, I called Mom from work to ask how everything was.

"He's doing great," she told me. "He may be home as early as next Monday."

On Thursday, however, there was a problem. The official report from the lab, where they sent a frozen section of lung tissue, conflicted with the preliminary findings taken during surgery; Dad's lung *was* infected by the cancer.

Mom was at a meeting in Poughkeepsie that afternoon, well over an hour away. It was the only time she was that far from Dad. When the doctors couldn't reach her, they decided to go ahead with the surgery since there was an operating room immediately available. They quickly explained the situation to Dad and began to prep him for the operation. But the suddenness of the situation was too much for Dad to handle. His heart went into an erratic condition. His pulse reached 180, and the doctors decided to delay the procedure.

Mom was so shaken by the news when my sister reached her at the meeting, that someone from Poughkeepsie had to drive her home, where Patrick was waiting to take her to the hospital. When she arrived at the hospital, Dad was back in his room and thankful to see her.

The doctors tried for an operating room for Monday but none was available. They had to wait for the next opening on Wednesday.

By that time I was on Christmas break from school and spent my non-working days in Highland Mills because I wanted to keep Mom company and be closer to the hospital. I told Mom that I would stay with her throughout the surgery on Wednesday and go to work only after we knew everything was okay.

• • •

On Wednesday morning, Mom arrived at the hospital before me, as I stopped at the bagel store for breakfast. The surgery was scheduled for 11:00, and Dad wasn't supposed to be wheeled down until 10:00, so when I arrived at 9:20, I thought I had plenty of time.

I rode up the elevator and walked towards Dad's room, but he wasn't there. I checked the room number. 506. It was the correct one. I feared something was wrong. What happened?

"They wheeled him down early," I heard a female voice

say from behind me. It was one of the nurses. "Your mother was here too, she's probably down in the waiting room now."

"Thank you," I told the nurse.

I hurried to the elevator. It was slow. I had to wait for them to wheel a woman off on the third floor. When I arrived on the first floor, I rushed to the waiting room and found Mom.

"What's going on, Mom? Is something wrong?"

"Nothing's wrong, Kev. They decided to take him early. I got here just in time to see him and wish him luck. He was asking for you."

He's probably worried that Mom will be alone. I want to let him know that I'm here.

"Can I get in to see him?" I asked Mom.

"There's Martha," Mom said, pointing to one of the nurses she had become friendly with. "I'll ask if she can do anything."

Mom went over to talk to Martha, and then motioned to me to join them.

"Martha is going to take you in to see him," Mom told me.

"Are you ready?" Martha asked.

"Yep."

We walked down the hall and through two sets of doors and Martha pointed at a wall full of hospital gowns. "You have to put on one of these gowns in order to go in," she said.

I had never worn a hospital gown before. Martha turned her head away from me as I struggled to put it on. When she turned back to me she said, "That's backwards." I took it off and tried again. When I got it right, we walked through another set of double doors and I saw Dad lying in a bed. Martha whispered, "Go ahead" and then left the room.

I thought he might be under the influence of some medication by this time, so I approached him like he was a senile man who might not know who I was.

"Dad, it's me, Kevin."

He smiled. "Kevin who?" he asked with a laugh.

He was fully aware of everything happening! They hadn't administered any anesthesia yet.

He took my hand as I reached his side.

"You look good in that outfit," he joked to me. "You should ask the nurse if you could keep the jacket."

On the other side of the bed, a male tech said, "Mr. Murphy, I don't know if you remember me, but I remember *you*. My name is Chris. I prepared you for your last surgery. I'm going to need to take a little blood."

It was as if they were friends. Perhaps they had a conversation last time.

"Chris, I'll give you five dollars to pretend you already did it," Dad joked with him as he rolled his head back toward me and smiled.

"Take mine instead!" I told Chris.

The tech poked him with a needle and began to draw his blood.

"I just wanted you to know that I was here, Dad."

"It's good to have you here," he told me.

"I'll be waiting outside with Mom until it's finished. Don't worry. I'll be with her the whole time."

Mom was such a concern to him. It was as if he thought that if she was comforted, everything else would work itself out: the surgery, the cancer, and the recovery. I was happy that I could ease his mind at least for that moment.

"Excuse me," another nurse interrupted us. "You're going to have to leave now," she said.

"Me or him?" Dad asked sarcastically from the bed.

I couldn't help but laugh. The others in the room, the techs, the nurses, all heard me laugh. They gave me strange looks. They weren't used to laughter in that room.

"Well, I think he should go, unless he wants to trade with you," the nurse told Dad.

I looked into Dad's eyes and thought about the goodness in his heart.

"I'll trade with you any day, Dad," I said to him. "Only I don't think I could ever do what you've done."

He gave me a sideways smile and said nothing.

"Well, let's leave that topic for another time," I said.

"Alright, we'll talk about it later," he told me. He was confident there was going to be a later.

"You'll do fine," I told him. "You've come too far not to. I'll be right outside if you need me."

"Okay," he said with a nod. "After the last one this should be easy, right?"

I nodded. Then I leaned over the bed and kissed him, and walked back through the double doors and back to Mom in the waiting room. We sat in the same far right hand corner as a week before. There were several other people in the room, but none in our corner.

I didn't want Mom to think about the surgery. I didn't want for her to envision this second viciousness, the second assault on Dad's body. Don't think about the reopening of the incisions, going through his tissues and chest cavity, inspecting his lung, slicing part of it off and removing it from his body. Think about something else, Mom. Dad will be sleeping, we will be here, the doctors will do the work and we will trust them. We'll find things to talk about, and soon it will be done. Everything will be okay. And there will be no more surgeries, no more cancer, no more decisions to make, no more waiting rooms, no more gowns.

I started to ask Mom questions about her life with Dad. Questions that children sometimes never get the chance to ask. What did they think life would be like together? How did they decide to have children? Did they always get along?

"We had some fights when we first got married, the first year or so," Mom told me. "It was all over little stuff, though. We worked it out."

"What about having kids?" I asked.

"As far as a family was concerned, we didn't plan things," Mom said. "We left it all up to God. I guess He thought we were ready for children almost right away though, because it didn't take long."

"What was that like?" I asked her as I moved my waiting room chair closer to hers.

"I'll never forget your father's reaction the first time Danny got sick," Mom said. "The doctor came to the house and gave us a prescription and Dad made a mad dash to the car and drove to the pharmacy a couple of blocks away. He waited for the prescriptions to be filled and then ran home as fast as he could. I noticed he was out of breath, but I didn't say anything."

"You mean he forgot to take the car home?" I asked with a laugh.

"Yeah, he left it at the pharmacy! He was so concerned

about little Danny. He didn't realize it until the next morning when I thought the car had been stolen!"

I smiled. Mom smiled. A fat woman and a small boy with a yoyo sat on a couch next to us. "What about Sharon?" I asked Mom.

"Yep, she was born the next year."

"I guess God wanted you to have kids."

"I guess so," Mom said as the boy played with his yoyo.

Mom went on to explain how they lived in a crowded one-bedroom apartment in Rosedale for more than three years. Mom and Dad slept on a pullout couch in the living room, while the two children shared the bedroom.

"And Dad, was he at IBM yet?" I asked.

"Yes, he started a couple of months before we got married," Mom told me. "He had to wear a suit to work and we had no money. So at the beginning of each year we financed four suits, two for summer and two for winter, and paid them off over the course of the year. By the end of the year the suits would be so worn out that we had to throw them away."

As the boy did tricks with the yoyo, Mom explained how Dad used to fix the machines at IBM. She said he was often on call and businesses would call in the middle of the night and she'd give him the phone and he'd ask them to hold on while he put the phone on his chest and tried to wake up. Many times she'd awaken an hour later and he'd be sound asleep with the phone still on his chest.

"I'd wake him up again," she told me, "and as soon as he hung up the phone it would start ringing again!"

I laughed. It sounded like something I would do. "You didn't work, did you?" I asked her.

"No, married women didn't work in those days. I left the FBI before we got married. But I remember one time when Dad was away that someone called with a problem in the middle of the night and I explained that Dad wasn't home. The person said he couldn't reach anyone at IBM, so I asked if he tried hitting the reset button in the back of the machine. Dad always asked them that first. The man tried it and it worked! So I guess you could say I filled in for Dad once in a while."

"How often did he go away?"

"He used to go away quite a bit for training seminars. I missed him so much," she told me as she pouted her lips. "One time he was going to California for two months, and I told him that he wasn't going without me. Not for two months! So Dad, Danny, Sharon, and I went to California. I loved the Sierra Nevada Mountains so much, we almost never came back."

"What about when he went by himself?" I asked.

"He'd call home every night. 'Ill—EE—vum' he used to say."

"What?"

"I-L-Y-V-M. He usually had a roommate and he was a little shy with his feelings around others. So he'd just say 'ill—EE—vum.' It stood for I love you very much."

I asked Mom about moving out of the tight confines and she explained that after saving money for a few years, they found a three-bedroom house they could afford in Queens Village in 1964. Dad painted the bigger of the two children's bedrooms pink, and the other one blue.

"I thought that girls had more of a need for big bedrooms," Mom told me.

"What about Patrick?"

"Well, he came along right after. So Dad got out his paintbrush again and repainted the pink bedroom blue and the blue bedroom pink. We bought bunk beds for the boys and they shared the bigger bedroom."

A nurse entered the waiting room. "Is there a Mrs. Fried here?" she asked. A woman in the front of the room raised her hand. "Follow me please," the nurse said. The woman put down her magazine and grabbed her pocketbook and followed the nurse.

Mom shook her head. "That's such a nervous feeling when they say that. You don't know where you're following them to. You don't know if it's good news or bad," she said as her eyes glazed over.

I shrugged my shoulders. "So, what was it like when you first moved to Queens Village?"

"It was great," Mom said. "Most of the neighbors were in the same boat as us, with young children and not much money. We became very close. The men all joined the Knights of Columbus, and the women were all involved in the church fundraisers and the schools."

"And me. What did you think about when I came along?"

She threw her right hand into the air. "We were shocked!" she said. "I had had an accident riding my bicycle several years before and we were told we couldn't have any more kids. But there you were."

The little boy dropped his yoyo and I bent over to pick it up and handed it to him. "And then we moved upstate?" I asked Mom.

"Yeah," she said. "It was a hard decision, but the Queens

Village group broke up. We were actually the last ones to leave in 1974. We always dreamed of having a big back yard for you guys to play in. So we saved our money and found the perfect property in Highland Mills and built a house."

"You fulfilled your dream, eh?"

"Yes. But do you remember how all our dreams were almost taken away?"

I was intrigued. "No, what do you mean?"

"Of course not," she said as she hit herself on the head. "You weren't even two years old yet." She went on to tell me the story of how we were visiting the house before moving in. Dad was going to Washington, DC that week for a seminar and had to catch a ride with a friend to the airport. There were two beautiful evergreens beside the house and Mom and Dad were planning to have the driveway circle around them. With all the kids packed into the family van, Mom and Dad saw our new neighbor, Mrs. Dwyer, walking on the street, and started to walk up to the street to talk to her.

"I reminded Dad that we didn't have much time," Mom told me. "So we decided to get into the van and drive up to the street and say a quick hello on the way out. Just after we pulled the van away, one of the evergreens fell, on the exact spot where the van had been."

"Wow," I said.

"I don't know if it was God's intervention or what. But you would have all been crushed if we didn't move the van at that instant. It would have crushed all of our dreams."

At noon, Mom and I went to the cafeteria for lunch. "Do you guys want anything?" I asked the woman and the yoyo boy as we got up. The woman raised her eyebrows at me as if I had broken an assumed code of silence between us waiting room neighbors. "Oh, thank you very much," she said with a smile. "We're just fine."

"Okay," I told her. "We'll be back soon. Don't let anyone take our chairs!"

Mom smiled at the woman. The boy looked up at me for a second, and then covered his face with his shirt.

As we walked to the cafeteria, Mom kidded with me, "You're so embarrassing."

"I like to think I'm polite," I said.

"Yeah, I guess you are," she said as we walked down the corridor.

The cafeteria special was fresh roast beef. We both ordered it. It was good. We continued to talk about the early years of living upstate. She told me about her and Dad going for bike rides around the neighborhood, to West Point to enjoy the scenery and have picnics, and for country drives to view the colors of the leaves in the fall. I remembered shoveling snow in the winter while Mom made hot chocolate, lighting firecrackers on the Fourth of July, and barbecuing on the back deck.

When we returned from lunch, the woman and the yoyo boy were gone. I hope they received good news. There were only a couple of people left in the waiting room. We took our same seats and I read the horoscopes to Mom and showed her some of the comics from the newspaper. We weren't quite as nervous as the first operation, but we were anxious for news.

At 2:30, Martha came into the waiting room and walked over to us.

"He's in recovery," she told Mom.

Mom grabbed my hand and pulled it to her lips and kissed my palm. I put my arms around her and leaned over to kiss her on the cheek.

"Can we see him?" Mom asked Martha.

"Well, I'm not supposed to let you," she said.

Mom pouted with her eyes. "But I'll take you in quickly," Martha added. "I have to warn you, though. He's not going to look very pretty. He just got out and they haven't cleaned him up yet. And I can only take you, Miriam. I'm sorry, but you can't both go."

I nodded my head. I understood. I didn't need to go. He didn't need to see me. And I didn't need to see him. I could wait. But Mom needed to see him.

She went. I waited.

Mom, please come back and tell me everything is okay. Be my fast food restaurant, my digital camera today. Tell me this is the finale. After today it all stops. It all gets better. Okay, recovery is a struggle and will take time, but everything will be fine. Come back soon and tell me all this and I will go to work. I'll be happy. I'll thank God. I won't worry any more. I'll count my blessings.

I waited in the corridor outside the waiting room. After fifteen minutes I saw Mom walking toward me in the hallway. I walked toward her and met her in the middle of the hall.

She nodded her head at me and smiled. "Everything's okay," she said. I gave her a hug. I didn't need to know anything else.

•   •   •

I stayed on Long Island the next three days while I was working, and on Saturday morning, Christmas Eve, I drove upstate to the hospital. Dad was in excellent spirits, and we had a nice conversation in the morning.

After going home for a few hours, I return to the hospital in the evening. Mom had been there all day, and Patrick joined her an hour before I came back.

We thought it best to get Dad walking again as soon as possible. He put up a fuss. "I'll try it a little later," he said.

"Dad, how can you come home for Christmas if you haven't been walking?" Pat asked him.

He must have been in an enormous amount of pain, because it took some convincing on our parts to get him motivated enough to try it. Finally, he put one arm around Patrick and one around me, and we walked out of the room and into the hallway. I could only imagine the excruciating pain it would have caused him to fall at that time. So Patrick and I gave each other a look and a nod, which implied "be careful". We had to make sure we held on to him securely, though not so tightly that we put pressure on his sore body.

We walked down the hall to the next room and then back to the nurses' desk, which was right in front of his room, where he rested for a minute while Mom introduced herself to the nurse on duty. We walked in the opposite direction until we reached the nurses' kitchen, about forty feet away, rested for a moment, turned back, and walked again to the nurses' desk. This was quite a workout for Dad, and when we got back to the nurses' desk, the two women were watching Dad to see how he responded to the exercise. He gave them no worries. With his arms around Patrick and I he leaned his body against the counter at the desk, and with perfect timing and eloquence he delivered the words, "Three beers please!" just as we reached the counter. It reminded me of a scene from a John Wayne movie, where John walks into a bar with two buddies after shooting up the town and demands a drink from the barkeep. Yeah, Dad was feeling okay.

That night Mom and I celebrated Christmas mass in the chapel. Dad had to stay in the room, but he watched the hospital broadcast of the mass.

Later we heard singing in the hallway. It was Sister Sheila and her friends singing carols for those who were spending Christmas in the hospital. I thought it was nice, but Mom and Dad saw it a different way.

"That's sad," Mom commented to Dad, as she looked at him with a frown.

"Why do you think it's sad, Mom?" I asked.

"Well, nobody wants to be here for Christmas. You're supposed to be home."

I didn't think about it that way. I was happy with Christmas as it was. My Christmas wishes were already answered. I didn't care about the celebration. I didn't care about seeing gifts under the tree with big letters on them: K, D, P, and S. I didn't care about our Christmas dinner. I was just happy to have a father.

Actually, we still held out hope the doctors would let Dad go home on Christmas Day. But we had no plans to celebrate. The family had agreed to postpone Christmas until the following week when we would exchange gifts and celebrate with a Christmas dinner on New Year's Day.

Mom, Dad, and I sat in the hospital and talked for a couple of hours about Christmases past, all remembering different things about them.

"Dad had a beard that he didn't shave off for about

three years," Mom told me. "On Christmas morning he came into the kitchen and started talking to me, but I didn't notice anything. He left the room laughing and I didn't know what he was laughing about and he wouldn't tell me."

Dad laughed. Just a small laugh. His body was too sore for much more than that.

"He came back a few minutes later and pointed at his lip," Mom continued. "He asked if I could see any swelling. I looked very closely and touched his face and told him that I didn't notice any swelling but that something seemed weird. Finally, he asked if there was anything on his face at all and I let out a scream when I realized he had shaved."

"How about the time you did the lights, hon?" Dad asked.

Mom broke out with hysterical laughing. "You know about that one, Kev?" she asked me through her laughter.

I had heard it many times before, yet I said, "Tell me about it."

"Well, decorating and undecorating for the holidays was something everyone shared in, but the lights were Dad's job," she started the story. "This one year, he was very busy at work and I decided it would be nice if I did it for him."

"Yeah, some help!" Dad said as he rolled his eyes. "She rolled five sets of lights all into one big ball!"

I laughed and Mom laughed. Dad laughed as much as he could. We reached such a volume that the nurse barged in and told us that we had to keep the noise down.

"So while I was so tired from work every night, I had to come home and untangle these lights. It took me three weeks!" Dad remembered.

"You'd come home from work and I'd make you a cup of tea and you'd work on the lights an hour each night!" Mom reminded him.

"That was the last time your mother ever touched the lights!" Dad told me.

•   •   •

At the hospital on Christmas Day, the doctors, although advising against it, gave Dad the option of going home. But he was feeling very weak and stayed in the hospital. We all went to see him and spend some time with him. As she had been doing for the previous two weeks, Mom stayed the entire day. Dad was allowed to leave the next day after two o'clock.

My father was a dignified man and insisted on leaving the hospital under his own terms. He was going to have his hair combed neatly, he was going to wear a shirt and pants, and he was going to walk out on his own power. He was strong, and these operations were not going to alter his spirit or his style. He was going to leave the hospital just as he had entered it two weeks earlier. He had fought this disease. He had gone through the chemotherapy, the radiation, and the mental struggles. He had survived the surgery, fell prey to further cancer, and survived a second surgery. He had battled all the demons that are cancer, and he had won. He was triumphant.

Dad had worn only loose sweat pants since the operation, and Mom couldn't imagine, given the location of some of the incisions, how he would be able to stand the pain of a buttoned pair of pants. She brought them anyway, but she was right, he couldn't wear them. He tried, but it was too painful.

When the nurse came by with the wheelchair, he said to her, "Listen, I've been up walking quite a bit this morning and I think I'll be okay. I don't think I need the chair."

"I would love to let you go," the nurse explained with a frown, "but I can't allow anyone to be released from this unit unless they are wheeled out."

"What if I said pleeeeease?" Dad kidded with the nurse.

"I'll tell you what," she succumbed. "I'll wheel you to the door, and then, if you want, I'll let you get up from the chair and walk out to the car. That's my best offer."

"Sold!" he shouted. "Get the car, Kev! We'll meet you outside!"

I ran down to the elevator smiling ear-to-ear. He was amazing. He was my hero. Nobody could approach his status in my little world.

For the record, my father waltzed out of Good Samaritan Hospital on December 26, 1994, with his hair combed to a shine, his face neatly shaved, and his body smelling fresh. He wore a light blue dress shirt tucked neatly into red sweat pants. Mom walked closely behind him, and in the background was a black woman in her forties, smiling brightly and shaking her head as she held on to a wheel chair.

TWELVE

Teenage Years

Mr. Strulovich is coming down the driveway to talk to Dad.

The Strulovichs are a family of Hasidic Jews. They are from the Kiryas Joel village nearby and have lived here for a couple of years, but their rabbi is angry with them because they are living so far from the temple, so I think they are going to have to move soon. We have always gotten along well despite our obvious lifestyle differences, and I even make money sometimes on Friday nights for turning on and off their electric and stove and things since they can't touch them after sundown. Recently they have begun keeping chickens and they let them roam free.

"Meester Murrr-phy," Mr. Strulovich says as he reaches Dad. "I'm sawddy to bodder you, but I am meezing vun of my cheeckeens. I zinc your dawk haft eaten it."

"Are you sure?" Dad asks.

"Jass."

Dad goes inside to find Patrick, who informs him that our dog, a big Siberian Husky and St. Bernard mix named Brandy, has been inside almost all day and couldn't have done *it. Dad explains this to Mr. Strulovich.*

A few days later, Mr. Strulovich visits again and makes the same claim. Dad checks for the dog, and again Brandy is inside.

"Sorry, I don't think it's our dog doing this," Dad tells him.

"But I'm chore eetz jour dawk."

"I'll make you a deal," Dad tells him. "I'll pay for the loss of the chicken nonetheless, provided that you put up some wiring to guard the chickens so that we don't have the problem of missing chickens again."

Mr. Strulovich doesn't take the money, but tells Dad that he is planning to put up a fence for the chickens soon. Meanwhile, Dad warns us to watch Brandy and make sure she doesn't venture into the neighbor's yard.

A week goes by without any incident, then, just as Mr. Strulovich is getting ready to put up the fence, he comes to the house again with another claim of chicken eating. This time, my father doesn't even check for the dog.

"Mr. Strulovich, I must insist that our dog doesn't eat kosher meat!" Dad jokes with him. "So she can't be eating your chickens."

With that, Brandy comes running around the corner, takes one look at Mr. Strulovich and lets out a bark. Out of her mouth flies a chicken feather.

• • •

I am in the bathroom throwing up. I drank Jack Daniels with Pat Hayes and Billy Dwyer while our parents were at a dinner with all the neighbors. This is the first time I ever drank more than one or two beers. Luckily, Mom and Dad won't be home for hours. I have time to get cleaned up.

"Kevin, what are you doing?"

"Mum? Hi!"

I guess it's later than I thought. Are they really home?

"What are you doing?"

"I dripped zomezing in da toila bowl."

"What do you have all over your sweatshirt?"

"Which switcher?"

"Did you have something to drink tonight?"

"Yeah, zorange juice. I dink I had too mush."

She disappears. I hear Mom and Dad talking in the next room but can't make out what they're saying.

Mom comes back and helps me to bed.

The next morning I have a headache. A bad headache. We go to church. Dad doesn't say a word to me and I try to tip-toe around the house the whole day and go to bed early.

Later in the week Dad and I talk about drinking and he tells me I am too young to drink. I get punished for several weeks and have to stay in the house, except for school, church, and school events. I don't argue with him, but I think he's wrong. I don't understand why he's making such a big deal out of it. Wasn't he ever a teenager?

• • •

Dad and I often watch Jeopardy at 7:00 and we compete for who can get the most answers correct. Today I found a trick. The same show is on at five o'clock on another channel!

I use my short-term memory to remember all the answers, and miss just two—intentionally—the entire first round of the show. Dad is amazed! He keeps shaking his head. "Miriam, you have to see our genius son!" he yells.

In the second round Skip gets a "Daily Double" in the category "Presidential Cabinets."

"Risk it all!" I scream. "I know my presidential cabinets like I know my own teeth!"

Dad looks at me intently.

"I'll risk a thousand, Alex," says Skip.

Alex Trebek reads the answer, "He was appointed the very first Secretary of the Navy."

"Ooooooh, what was his name, Dad?" I pretend.

Then I really lay it on thick. "You know," snapping my fingers, "he was wounded at the Battle of Brandywine."

"Brandywine?" Dad scratches his head.

I know I have time 'cause Skip doesn't know the answer.

Still snapping my fingers. "John Adams appointed him! Geez, I can't remember...oh yeah, Stoddert! Benjamin Stoddert!" I yell.

"Three seconds, Skip," Alex says.

One, two, three. "Any guess? Sorry Skip," Alex informs him. "Wounded at the battle of Brandywine and appointed by John Adams, it was Benjamin Stoddert."

Dad begins to laugh. I know exactly what he is laughing about. He doesn't know how I did it, but he knows my new-found intelligence is not quite authentic. He laughs all the way through Final Jeopardy.

• • •

Short order cook, $400/week. Nope. Stable help, $7/hour. Nah. Models and actors wanted, up to $3000 per week! Hmmm.

"How 'bout this one, Dad? Sales managers wanted. Several openings for highly motivated workers in direct sales. Up to

$1500 dollars per week."

"Notice the 'up to' part. $1500 per week sounds too good to be true, Kev."

I go for an interview with them anyway and find out their product is basically glorified vacuum cleaners that sell for $1395 apiece. They convince me that I would be a good sales-person and introduce me to another guy who made a lot of money with them. Dad is quite skeptical about the job. "I tried something just like that when I was your age and never made any money," he tells me.

"Yeah, but this is gonna be soooooo easy, Dad," I tell him as I think about how much money I will have to buy beers and go for spring break. "I can make so much more like this," I insist.

"I think it's a very risky venture and you really shouldn't take the risk. You should find a different job with an hourly wage," he says.

"You're always trying to keep me back!" I tell him as I insist that I can make the money they advertised.

Finally, he stops trying to discourage me.

Two months later, I have sold just one vacuum cleaner and made $150 along with two free lunches. I have no money to go out with my friends and drink beers and go to Six Flags and all the other fun stuff.

I ask Dad if I can borrow a few dollars for gas and food. He gives me some money. He doesn't rub it in—the fact that the job didn't work out and he was right. I feel guilty when I spend his money to buy beer and party with friends.

Eventually, I take Dad's advice and find another job with an hourly wage.

THIRTEEN

A Sigh of Relief

I had visions of my father dancing around the living room when he returned home from the hospital. Though I knew it would be a long recovery, I thought he'd at least be able to move around, that he'd smile and talk with us as if he were healthy.

These things were not to be when he first came home. The trip home itself consumed much of his energy. He was too tired to even enjoy the scenery, which was one of his favorite things about living in Orange County. There was a "Welcome Home John" sign on the Littmann's driveway, and he gave a brief smile when he saw it, but he couldn't manage much more than that.

When we got inside he stopped downstairs to say hello to Sharon, Jamie, and Benjamin. They had been living downstairs for several months since Sharon had separated. The kids made cards that read, "Get well soon, Grandpa," and "We love you, Grandpa." The cards made him smile. He loved his grandchildren. From putting Jamie to sleep by reading her stories, to sitting Benjamin next to him in the garage when he did some carvings, to visiting with Daniel on Long Island, he stayed involved with his grandchildren.

Dad asked me to bring the cards upstairs for him, and then I helped him walk the two sets of stairs to the living room. Halfway up, he took a rest and struggled for air. He was used to having two fully functioning lungs, and would now have to get used to a new way of breathing.

"Now I can empathize with Grandma," he commented, referring to the difficult time Grandma Cronin had climbing the stairs with only one-half of a lung. By the time we got upstairs, he was exhausted.

Physically, we tried to comfort him, but nothing we could do was enough. No matter what position he sat or lay in, he was in pain. He insisted he was better off sleeping on the pull-out couch in the living room, so I brought angular pillow heads from another couch and stuffed a couple of regular pillows in front of them to make for a smooth incline. But he still wasn't comfortable.

Mom slept on the couch with him while their bedroom remained empty for the night. Though she wanted to squeeze him and hold him as tightly as she could, she had to resist the temptation out of concern for his sore body.

• • •

The first week of recovery went by quickly. Every morning a nurse came to the house to check on Dad and change the dressing on his wounds. But he didn't show much improvement the first couple of days, and on Wednesday I had to leave him to go to Long Island and work. I crossed my fingers that he would show some improvement by the time I saw him again Saturday morning.

I went straight to my parent's house from work around

five am that Saturday, and slept there. By the time I woke up it was afternoon. Dad wasn't in his room. I checked the kitchen and the living room. No Dad. Mom was on the phone in the kitchen and I interrupted her. Was everything all right?

"Where's Dad?" I asked Mom in a concerned tone.

"Hold on one second," she spoke into the phone. "He went downstairs to look at his carousel horse," she said to me with a wink.

"Really?"

I didn't believe it! Just that he could walk down the stairs on his own was amazing! I went into the garage and there he was sitting on his stool looking over his masterpiece.

It was nice to see him back in the garage where he had built an entire workshop on one side and left the other side for Mom to park her car in the winter. He had filled the floor space on his side with large machines such as a band saw and a drill press and acquired numerous tools and other "handyman stuff" over the years to fill the cabinets over his workbench. Gradually he had acquired the tools and knowledge for almost any circumstance. Most of the neighbors had realized this and knew where to go for advice or to borrow something.

"How are you feeling, Dad?" I asked him from the doorway of the garage.

"Hey, Kev. Actually, I'm feeling quite a bit better than a week ago. I heard you come in this morning. How are you?"

"I'm fine. I'm just so happy to hear that you're feeling well! How's the horse?"

He put his hand on the horse's head and gave it a pat.

"Just a few finishing touches to make," he said. "Then the painting."

"What color are you going to paint it?" I asked as I walked toward his masterpiece and patted her.

"Colors, you mean," he said to me. "I'm not sure yet which colors. I want it to have a feminine look. But I may not do the painting myself. I don't have enough confidence in my painting abilities yet. I want it to come out just right. I may give it to Pete's wife for the painting, she's really good."

I smiled. He nodded his head and smiled. This is what I had looked forward to. Seeing him happy. He deserved it.

"Well, you look good," I said.

He winked at me. I put my arms out and gave him a hug. Not too much of a squeeze, not yet. But a well deserved hug.

He was back.

• • •

On New Year's Eve, Dad was feeling well enough to have company at the house. The Littmanns and the Bensons came over to help ring in 1995. I usually went out with friends, but contemplated staying home.

"We'd love to have you," Dad told me. "But it's not necessary that you stay. Go do what you want, have fun, and be safe. Just make sure you're back New Year's Day for our Christmas celebration."

So I went out with friends to Hunter Mountain, but called home after midnight. I had never missed wishing my parents a Happy New Year, whether I was with Grandma and Grandpa Cronin as I had been when I was very young,

or whether I was at a friend's party when I became older.
This night I waited a half-hour at the pay phone in Slope's
to make the phone call.

"1995 will be a much better year than 1994!" I
screamed to my mother through the deafening noise in the
club. "I'm very confident about that!" In the background
I could just make out the sounds of my neighbors talking
loudly and laughing with Dad.

I drove home the next morning and we opened our
Christmas gifts after our family's traditional Christmas breakfast: eggs, hash browns, bacon, sausage, and English muffins.

I gave Dad a group of books planned to coincide with
his progression. I had already given him *Politically Correct
Bedtime Stories* for some easy, humorous reading in the hospital. The next books in the line were *The Chamber* by John
Grisham and Tom Clancy's latest *Debt of Honor*. The last
book in my gift package was *The History of the IRA*, a book
that needed to be read slowly and accurately. Dad had
already read a thick book on Irish history. I figured that
when I saw him reading the IRA book, it would mean he
was nearly recovered.

We had our traditional Christmas dinner that night: filet
mignon. At the dinner table, I felt thankful we were all
there as Dad led us in saying grace:

Bless us, O Lord
For these thy gifts which we are about to receive
From thy bounty
Through Christ, our Lord
Amen

"Mom and I are very happy that you have all joined us this year. It's great to be here," Dad continued.

Nobody moved. The food waited. It could wait. We didn't care about the food. There could have been no food; we wouldn't have cared. Burned filet mignon, raw eggs, whatever. It wouldn't have mattered. It was Christmas, or at least, it was *our* Christmas celebration. And we were experiencing Christ's gift in its purest form: Life.

"Here's to health," Danny said as he lifted up his glass.

"And to more Christmases together," I added as everyone around the table touched their glasses together.

Dad tried a piece of filet mignon, but couldn't eat more than a couple of bites. He also tried some corn and a roll with butter, and although during his illness he often had to excuse himself from the table after eating only a little bit, he felt well enough to sit at the table and participate in the conversations.

Later that night he threw up. He had to get used to food again, and to the new feelings in his esophagus. It was going to take some time.

• • •

It was nice to be home for vacation for a couple of weeks as Dad was recovering. He made obvious improvements each week.

The second week after the surgery, I noticed him reading a bit. He was looking at various books and magazines in search of the perfect color combination for his carousel horse. Later in the week he spent a bit of time on the computer. The next week he began going to H&R Block to update Mom's computers and help her with the payroll.

And eventually, he made the finishing touches on his carousel horse.

One morning I drove him to H&R Block and we talked on the way.

"When do you think they'll let you drive, Dad?" I asked.

He sat in the passenger seat looking out the window. "Oh, I think it will be a long time. I can't even imagine driving right now," he said as he turned his head to look at me. "I mean, I can walk fine, but you can't imagine how difficult it is to get around sometimes, with the soreness and the breathing and all."

"No kite flying or throwing boomerangs anytime soon, then?"

He smiled. "No, it will be a while," he said as he turned back to look out the window at the scenery. "But it'll come back. It's just going to take some time."

I noticed the long, fancy, leather jacket he was wearing. It was the first leather jacket he had ever owned. He looked good in it, and it made his thin body look a bit fuller. Mom bought him the jacket at the end of the previous winter. She said it was about time he had something nice to wear for winter. It was a treat, like Mom's mink coat and their 25th anniversary cruise on the QE2. But I had the feeling that they would start treating themselves to nice things more often. I was trying to get them to take a trip to Ireland. They were hoping to do it next summer.

Dad continued to look out of the window as I drove, just like I looked out the window years ago when I was a small kid and he drove me places. Funny, it's the little things that you remember. Those are the most important. I remember him being there at Little League games and school plays. I remember how he used to laugh at me when I said funny things that I didn't know were funny as a child. When I looked at him strangely he would stop laughing because he didn't want to hurt my feelings. And I remember all the little things he did with me, all the times he helped me. Some people affect our lives so greatly in such simple ways. They may never even know it—I wonder if he knew the full fruit of what he did for me.

There is a certain amount of regret we feel as adults. We finally realize things we didn't appreciate as kids, things we missed out on. We become aware of the hurt our actions may have caused and we feel guilty, but this is just the way kids are. Guilt and questioning are pointless, as useful as being angry at the sun for setting each day. It's just the nature of things.

I once read a quote from the golfer Bobby Jones. He said, "Play the ball as it lies". And he wasn't talking about golf. He was referring to life's obstacles, and to life's regrets. Dad was playing the ball as it lay all the way through his battle, and I tried to do the same. Neither one of us could go back. We could only try to make the best of what was in front of us.

• • •

Dad called Mr. Littmann the day of the Super Bowl to ask if he wanted to watch the game with us. Bruce Littmann had been coming over for a number of years to watch the Super Bowl, since he was the only male in his house among three girls.

Dad and Bruce had a great relationship. Although the rest of the world was unaware, they often solved world problems, at least theoretically. Even when they disagreed, they realized that their differences were battles of ideas, not of people. Often, Dad would be on his way home from somewhere and see Bruce getting the mail or doing something else at the bottom of his driveway. These chance meetings usually turned into long conversations, sometimes into demonstrations of a new "toy" one of them had purchased, and often turned into plans of a double date with their wives, such as a movie or dinner.

Bruce walked in less than five minutes into the game just as Jerry Rice was scoring the 49ers' second touchdown. He brought a can of peanuts with him, but Dad couldn't eat any. His wife later joked with him, "The man just had surgery and you brought peanuts?"

Mr. Littmann had been running around all weekend and had to go to work in the morning, so he was tired. He kept falling asleep in the chair. Dad and I laughed and shouted, "Hey, Bruce!" a few times when he nodded off. Each time, Mr. Littmann opened his eyes quickly and pretended that he wasn't asleep. Dad and I laughed.

What made everything so great was that Dad was feeling really well. He smiled and laughed and talked that night and for the whole week before it, more than he had smiled and laughed since before he became sick. Just by looking at him, anyone could tell how well he was doing. The color had come back to his face. There was a spark in his eye. There was an air of triumph in his step. He was well on his way to recovery. Even a fool could see that.

When Mr. Littmann left that night, he too must have had a good feeling about Dad's progress and he must have been thinking that he would be back to watch many future

Super Bowls with his good friend. But in fact, that would be the last time they would enjoy each other's company.

•   •   •

After the Super Bowl, I told Dad I was thinking about playing a racquetball tournament the next weekend and that I might not be home if I did well. I had given up racquetball for two months, but had worked out my rustiness after a few days of hitting the ball earlier in the week.

"I don't mind if you don't come home," Dad told me. "I appreciate that you've spent a lot of time at home lately. I know it's the heart of racquetball season. I don't want to see you miss any more than you already have."

So the next weekend, I went to the tournament. It was at the BQE club in Woodside, so I stayed in Long Island Friday night. Saturday night I called Mom and Dad to say I had made it to Sunday and wouldn't be home at all that weekend.

"How's Dad?" I asked Mom.

"He's sleeping," she told me. "He's been having headaches."

"Headaches?"

"Yeah, very bad ones," she sighed. "You remember years ago, he had migraine headaches?"

"I remember," I said.

Many years earlier Dad had terrible migraine headaches that came and went, but after treatment they eventually went away for good. I prayed that they hadn't come back to him again, especially at this time. He was already coping with so much pain. I couldn't bear to think of him dealing with anything else.

Nonetheless, I reasoned that the headaches now were probably from lack of food. Whatever the cause, I was sure it was unrelated to the cancer, and minuscule compared to it. Even if he had to deal with some headaches, he had already proven that pain was no match for his will.

"We went to the doctor today," Mom told me. "He gave Dad some medication to take for the headaches. We'll see how that works. I can't stand to think of him in more pain," she said.

"I'll pray that it will go away, Mom."

"I wish the doctors could give the headaches to me," she said. "He's been through so much already."

I would take the headaches, too. Take away the pain. Leave him alone, all you devils of pain. Leave him alone!

"Well," I told Mom, "you tell Dad I'll be home next weekend and he should make sure he's feeling better."

"Okay, I'll tell him," she said.

During the tournament, one of the guys from Pennsylvania came over to me while I was warming up to inquire about my recent whereabouts. "Where have you been lately, Murf? You've missed some good stops."

"Actually, my father has cancer and I've been spending my free time with him," I told him.

"I'm very sorry to hear about the cancer. At least it's good that you have your priorities in order," he said. "How is he doing?"

"Much better now, thanks. He's actually having a few headaches this week, but overall he's doing really well. He's on his way to a full recovery."

I played the tournament with a renewed enthusiasm. It had nothing to do with my enthusiasm for the game itself. It was the enthusiasm of thankfulness. I was thankful to have my family. Thankful that Dad had come through.

Actually, the few weeks directly following his surgery, in January 1995, were some of the happiest of my life. I thought everything was good. I enjoyed everything I did. Dad was getting a second chance at life. I was getting a second chance to know him. This time, I would appreciate him more. I would see the things he did for me and openly acknowledge them. I would fish with him again, something we had stopped doing since I was a teenager and became too cool to fish with my father. I would go places with him. I would call him on the phone and have conversations. I would openly discuss my problems with him. And I would never miss another opportunity to hug him.

I sat there, at the tournament, recovering from the emotional roller coaster ride that cancer gives to every family it infects: ups, downs, screams, laughs, fears, thrills.

And, as if I hadn't learned my lesson before, I made another premature assumption: I thought that the ride was over.

FOURTEEN

Becoming an Adult

Saturday afternoon, a few months after coming back from flight school in Texas.

"What are you doing today, Kev?" Dad asks me as he's buttering his toast.

"Not sure. Why, you had something in mind?" I ask as I pull out a box of waffles from the freezer.

"Well, the club purchased some wood and it's being delivered today at Ralph Rogo's garage. We could really use an extra hand offloading it from the truck and stacking it in the garage. It'll just be a couple of hours. Want to give us a hand?"

I put the waffles in the toaster. I wouldn't have even thought about this question several years ago, I would have just told him I had other things I wanted to do.

"Sure, I'll give you a hand," I tell him. "You think we can be back for the football game at four o'clock?"

"I can make sure that we are," he says.

We meet the other carvers at Ralph's house while we wait for the flatbed to arrive. Dad introduces me to his woodcarving friends. "Everybody this is Kevin, my son!" he tells the four carvers who were there to help offload the wood. "*He volunteered to give us a hand today.*"

The carvers seem to respect me instantly. They all want to shake my hand. I can tell they have a lot of respect for Dad.

It takes about ninety minutes for us to unload the wood and stack it inside. After we're done Dad asks me if I would like a beer. It's the first time he has ever offered me to have one with him, so I'm a little taken back.

"*Sure, I'll have one,*" *I tell him.*

We relax in Ralph's back yard and talk with the other guys and to each other. I don't feel like a son, more like a friend.

As I am about to reach my twenties, Dad and I have become buddies.

• • •

I am home from college for a few days. Dad went out to the store. The telephone rings.

"*Kev, I locked my keys in the car. Could you do me a big favor and get my spare set and bring them to me?*"

"*Sure, no problem,*" *I tell him.* "*Where are they?*"

"*I keep them in my memento box on top of my dresser, you know the one?*"

"*Yeah, I know it. I'll get them and bring them to you.*"

I walk into his room, find the box and open it. I've never looked inside this box before. The keys are at the top. I recognize a few articles underneath.

A wedding picture of him and Mom.

A congratulations letter from IBM.

A baseball card of me from baseball camp.

A newspaper article from a game I pitched.

A program from one of Sharon's dance recitals.

A photograph of Patrick at his First Communion.

A test report of Danny's SAT scores.

This is what he keeps in here? This is a collection of his most prized possessions in life? These are the things he treasures?

* * *

The Littmanns are over for dinner and have brought their first completed "memory book" of Cape Cod, the book their rotating weekly guests and renters sign before they leave.

I look through the entries from our family and see a lot of pages filled up by Dad's handwriting. I can see that he enjoyed his times there and I can see that sharing that enjoyment with the family was important to him:

1988: "Night swims at the pond. Scaring Dianne. Moby Dick's fish & chips. Lobster-Lobster-Lobster. Hammer Dulcimers at P-Town. Sailing. Flying. Mason & Sullivan (clocks) in S. Yarmouth...Memories of the wonderful, tranquil early morning breakfasts at the pond. Mary Ellen's décor. Hectic 'tourist' type shopping. Fixin' things. P-Town and the people there (well, <u>some</u> people). Kite-flying at the beach. New box kite. Being with the family. Patrick next year? Planning it better for next year!"

1989: He makes an advertisement for himself, "Woodcarving, things fixed, other services available: contact John Murphy" and below it draws an empty box and writes "Space available. See your ad here!" He then goes on to warn other renters, "The Chinese are wrong...this is definitely the year of the mosquito."

1990: He says: "Once again, it's a pleasure to be here… this time with Grandma Cronin and Patrick (again). But also joined by Mom & Dad Murphy. Nice surprise to have them. Miss the others, of course!"

He goes on that year to tell of the daily excursions of a kayaking expedition he made with Patrick to Jeremy Point:

Day #1 "On our preparation runs on Long Pond, many townspeople cheer us on from the shores, we think."

Day #2 "To round out our experience, we now tackle the Ponds Gull & Higgins. We discover another pond connected to Higgins, which is unknown according to any maps produced by Bruce. We name it "Bills Pond" because I lost two dollar bills from my shirt pocket here."

Day #3 "Our expedition suffers a severe setback today, as we oversleep & decide to succumb to a late bacon & egg breakfast"

Day#4 "We reach the end of Grand Island about 2pm, only to discover that Jeremy Point is gone!! Missing!! The water where it should be is very turbulent; leading us to suspect it has sunk! We must return and report this to the authorities immediately! But first, we beach the kayaks to enjoy a leisurely swim and a lunch of RITZ (the original) crackers and warm seltzer. Finally, we launch to report our amazing findings. Near catastrophe almost engulfs us as I, in my anxiety to install my spray skirt, am nearly pulled into the abysmal eddies of what was once Jeremy Point! Only the skills developed by constant practice in the confines of Long Pond save me as I paddle skillfully out of harm's way…On the return trip, the sun beats down unmercifully. We beach at Great Beach Hill to escape its unforgiving rays, only to be besieged by the GREEN HEADED

FLIES. Unable to defeat the enemy (without fly swatters), we flee back to the sea. God is with us, as the 'partly cloudy' part of the forecast takes effect"

1991: He adds to the kayaking story stating "We return to check on Bruce's preposterous suggestion that Jeremy Point will resurface when the "Tide" is out. We check all the nearby harbors and inlets and can find no sign of the "Tide", nor any similarly named ship. It must be out. With the Tide out, we look for Jeremy Point. It is still not there, after nearly a year!!"

• • •

Dad, Grandpa, and I are at the golf driving range in Monroe on a summer evening. Grandpa picked up golfing when he turned 70, and at 88 is now an avid golfer and often shoots a score lower than his age for 18 holes. But I think this is the first time Dad has hit a golf ball.

I played for a while back in ninth grade, but haven't played the last several years. I'm happy to come to the range to hit the ball, but moreover, it is an interesting feeling to be on a three-generation men's outing. I don't know how many opportunities like this one a person can get, so I treat it as being special.

Dad tries hitting a few balls and none of them go very far. He's a good sport but I can see he is getting frustrated.

Grandpa says, "It's your stance, John" and shows him a better one.

"I wanna make just one good shot and look like a pro!" Dad tells us.

When Grandpa's lesson is over, Dad steps up to the ball

and swings. "Wow! Look at that one!" I shout to them.

Dad looks back at me with an excited look on his face. "Where is it?"

I raise my left hand to my brow in the golfer's salute to indicate I am watching the ball high up in the air. The ball really went just thirty feet, but had stopped rolling by now and I am certain neither one saw it. Surely they'll get a good laugh out of it when I point to the ball and reveal the truth, I figure.

Now Dad has a boyish expression, proud of himself for hitting a good shot. Grandpa says "How 'bout that, John! I knew you could do it. After all, you're my son!"

I think about how it would make me feel to be in his shoes, and if he were in Grandpa's. I think about what I had heard one time, that it had taken them a long time to get close to each other because in the years when Dad was young and learning who his family was, Grandpa was away in the army. I think about the specialness of this time together and about the two of them as father and son, how they have become close just like Dad and I. I think about us enjoying a time like this together in 20 years when I have a family. I can't tell them the truth about the ball.

"It's coming down now," I tell them.

"Where?" Dad asks.

"Just landed past the sign that says 160," I say.

"Wow 160 John, that's some shot!" Grandpa screams.

"Yeah, well, I think you were right," Dad says. "This is a much better way for me to stand."

"You're a good student," Grandpa says.

"Well, I have a great teacher."

"Yeah, but it's you that hit the ball."

Dad hits another one. Whack!

"Another good one John!" Grandpa yells. "Look at that, you're getting the hang of it."

"Well, that's not 160 but it's pretty good," Dad says.

"You know what else I do John, let me show you something else you can try too. I take my arm..."

I go back to my own ball and leave Dad and Grandpa to themselves. This is a moment for them.

FIFTEEN

~⚡~

There Was No Parachute

It was Tuesday at 6:30. I was driving to the supermarket to get some food when my pager beeped. I reached into my pocket, pulled it out, and looked at the number. I was pretty sure it was Danny's work number with a "911" at the end, indicating it was urgent. Dianne was a few months into her second pregnancy, so I thought she needed something while Dan was stuck in his office. I was only five minutes from their house and thought about heading straight there, but I was already making the turn into the supermarket and there was a public phone there so I decided to call first.

I parked the car, walked to the phone, and dialed the number.

"Hello."

"Dan?"

"Kevin. Where are you?"

There was an alarming tone to his voice.

"I'm...I'm calling you from a phone booth...near a supermarket."

"Dad's in the hospital."

The hospital? I closed my eyes and allowed my head to fall backwards, as if preparing for a knockout blow.

"What's wrong?" I asked, fearing the answer.

"They found another tumor," Dan said. "In his brain."

I suddenly remembered what the book mentioned in September about metastasis and how cancer can spread to other body parts.

My heart fell out of my chest.

Brain cancer. The words were lethal. It sounded incurable. Does anybody survive brain cancer?

I looked for something to throw or to hit. There was only my pager and my wallet in my pockets, and neither one would fly as far as I needed them to.

Rip the phone out of the damn wall and throw it! Throw it through the window of the store; break all the panes of glass! Make all the customers scream and run away in horror!

I stamped my feet with force on the pavement below. I jumped and landed with all my might trying to break through the pavement. A woman with long, hanging earrings and Purdue chickens in her shopping cart gave me a look as if to say I should calm down. Come over here, lady, I'll rip those earrings out of your ears and make you bleed! Tell me to calm down?

A man with a limp walked toward me and stopped a few feet away. Was he going to wait for this phone? I gave him a vicious stare and crinkled my nose and showed him my teeth like a dog in a growl. Go away, mister! Don't wait for this phone!

I returned to the conversation. "What happened, Dan?" I asked him, desperate for some information.

"I'm not really sure. Sharon just called me a few minutes ago. I haven't talked to Mom and Dad yet."

"This sucks!"

"I know. I can't believe it," Dan said.

What can they do now? Can they get rid of it?

"Do they operate for brain cancer?" I asked Danny.

"Sometimes, I think it depends on the type," he said. "I'm going to try to call Dad at the hospital and put us both through on conference call. So hold on, okay?"

"Okay."

What I didn't know at the time was that Dad's headaches had gotten much worse since I last spoke to my parents two nights earlier. In the morning they had gone for a CATSCAN. In the afternoon, they were in Dr. Young's office when he received the results from the hospital over the telephone. Mom and Dad noticed that Dr. Young's voice became soft and his eyes moist. When he hung up the phone, he gave a sad look to my parents.

"There are tumors in the brain," he said. "I'm sorry, I don't know what happened."

Mom grabbed Dad's hand and began to cry. They hugged and cried. They pleaded with the doctor that it must be wrong. It couldn't be true. They cried and held hands all the way to the hospital. They cried and cried. Mom cried. Dad cried.

There was a medical team that met them at the hospital. They checked Dad into a private room. They showed him the pictures. It wasn't just a tumor. There were multiple tumors. They were all over his brain. Left side and right side. They were inoperable. There wasn't much the doctors could do now. They began administering steroids to try to shrink the tumors and control the growth, but the situation was basically hopeless. They said he might have a week to live, or a month, maybe a little more. The vicious invader had given no warning.

Danny connected us on the conference call. "Dad, it's Dan and I have Kevin on the line with us," he said.

"Hi, Dad, I'm here too," I said.

"Hi. How are you guys?" Dad asked us.

How are we? What does he mean, how are *we*? I let Dan take over the conversation.

"We just heard, Dad. How are you?" Dan asked.

"I can't lie," Dad said. "I'm very disappointed."

"Us too. How do you feel?" asked Dan.

"Well, they've relieved some of the pain with the steroids. It works very quickly. I've been in so much pain. It had really gotten unbearable."

"Have the doctors mentioned anything about treatment?"

"Not too much. They're just concentrating on relieving the pain right now. They're taking a look at where everything is and we'll try to come up with a plan from there."

I couldn't speak. It was like my mouth was glued shut.

"Hey, the conference call thing is pretty neat," Dad said. "First time I've used it. It's pretty cool to have all three of us on the same phone from three different places. Kev, you're there, right?"

I was trying to control myself. My right hand was closed in a fist. People were walking by with their shopping carts. What kind of people were these?

I tried to compose myself. Dad was composed.

"I'm here Dad. I just don't know what to say," I told him.

"Me too," he said. "Let me put Mom on, she wants to talk to you guys."

Mom came on the phone and commented how proud she was of our family. She said it was a nice feeling that we were all together so soon after hearing the news. Patrick and Sharon were already at the hospital with them.

Some months later, Mom was encouraged by a few people to bring a lawsuit against the hospital for malpractice. She had mixed emotions about it. I know that one of the doctors sent a sympathy card after the funeral, and Mom didn't send him a thank you note like she did to the other people who sent cards. But in the end, when thinking about the doctors, she kept coming back to one thing. That night at the hospital, she remembers the doctors wiping tears from their faces as they tried to explain the possibilities. Dad had become their friend.

I don't believe other doctors would have made things any different. Bad things sometimes happen in life, and we must deal with them. Just because we've lost out doesn't mean we have to find someone to pay for it. It doesn't make it better. Dealing with it makes it better. Talking about it makes it better. Writing about it makes it better. Becoming a better person because of it makes it better. Even if there was something the doctors could have done, I don't want to know. Not anymore. It wouldn't help Dad. It wouldn't help me.

It was God's decision. To sue would have been like saying that God intended for my father to live, but was overpowered by a doctor's mistake. The God I believe in would not let that happen.

• • •

On Saturday, I drove to the hospital with Sharon to see Dad. When we walked past the waiting room, the sanctuary of all the hopes and fears I had experienced over the past several months, I cringed.

Dad was sleeping when we walked into the room. He woke for a few brief seconds and gave us a very soft "Hello". But he fell right back to sleep. We decided not to stay.

The steroids had helped him to feel much better, relieving the pain from the pressure the tumors had been putting on his skull. But the doctors had also found a mark on his adrenal gland, and were concerned that it might be an additional tumor.

I went back to the hospital later in the evening. Again, Dad was sleeping when I walked into the room. I was content to sit next to his bed and look at him. I thought about all the pain and stress he went through with the operations. Was it all for nothing? If he doesn't make it, was it all a waste? No, it was a fight. And a damn good one. It was full of courage and love. It was inspiring. And that's the most anyone can do. And it wasn't over yet. There was always a chance. As long as we had our family, as long as we had God, there was always still a chance. I wasn't giving up.

Dad woke up after a few minutes. He told me that Mom was at the chapel attending mass and he turned the television to the hospital broadcast of the mass. Dad commented that the audio was very poor on the broadcast. I reminded him that Sharon and I had stopped by earlier. He told me that he recalled us stopping by, and that his nap had made him feel much better.

Then he looked into my eyes. "How are *you* doing?" he asked.

Don't ask me that, Dad. I'm doing shitty and I don't want to tell you. It won't help you.

"I've been very sad, Dad," I said.

A long silence. My eyes started to water. He reached his hand out and put it around mine and told me something I'll never forget.

"It's part of life, Kev."

I nodded my head. He squeezed my hand.

"You have to deal with these things," he told me. "It won't be the last time for you."

I nodded again and wet my lips. They were dry, cracking.

"Let's not give up hope yet," Dad said to me.

I shook my head with confidence. "Oh, I haven't. I have a lot of hope. I'm hoping for the best. You deserve the best."

He moved his only free hand to wipe his eyes and lifted his head off the pillow and raised his brow. "Hmmmm?"

"I said you deserve the best, Dad! The absolute best. Nothing but the best for you."

"Thank you," he said. "You're a good son."

Was I? Did I do good things? Don't good sons obey? I didn't always obey. Are good sons allowed to hate you for punishing them when they're young? Do good sons tell you that they don't want to go fishing with you anymore because they're too cool? Do they lie to you about what they do with their friends when they are teenagers?

But these weren't the things he remembered about me. They happened yes, but he brushed them aside as adolescent behavior. Instead he remembered taking me to the Hall of Fame, going fishing together, and watching Jeopardy with me on weeknights. He remembered visiting a Navy recruiter with me, remembered our golf outing with Grandpa, and remembered when I came home from Texas and how we hugged on the driveway. He remembered how much I prayed that he would beat the cancer. And if these would be his last days, I was going to make sure that his last memories of me were good ones.

"You're a good father," I told him. "I'm really proud of you. I'm proud of what you've done in life. I'm proud of how you've fought this thing."

We sat silent again, just holding each other's hands. The mass was almost over. Mom would be back soon. "I love you," he told me.

Those may be the three most powerful words when used together, but are often brushed away with a quick "Yeah, me too" or "I love you, too." I didn't respond like that. I looked at Dad and thought about the words and what they really meant.

When I was a little boy I had often asked my parents to explain to me what love was. They tried to explain it to me as best they could, but it was never to my satisfaction. I kept asking in my pre-teen voice, "Is it kind of like liking someone a lot?" They would answer, "Sort of...but there's more to it than that."

I struggled to get the words out. "You and Mom...mean more to me...than anything in the world." His eyes looked up at mine, his head resting on the pillow. "You know, I have never thought...that you would do anything *but* recover from this. I'm going to keep thinking that way."

"I appreciate your concern," he said, "but I'll be fine no matter what happens. We'll all keep praying. It's not in our hands anymore. It's up to God."

I wiped my eyes.

"But listen to me, carefully," he said. "Mom is the one who needs the most help. She's having a hard time. Help *her*. That's what you can do for me."

So selfless.

I would help Mom. After he was gone, I would stay up late nights and talk to her about Dad. I would hold hands and pray with her. I would buy her books about heaven and the afterlife. I would take her on a trip to Ireland in the summer. And I would put together a collection of memories of Dad's life for her to keep.

"You know, it's going to be Valentine's Day," I said to Dad. "You want me to get something for you to give Mom?"

"Wow, Valentine's Day. You know, with everything happening, I almost forgot about Valentine's Day. Would you get a plant for Mom and give it to her from me? I prefer plants instead of flowers because they last much longer."

"What kind?"

"Anything you pick out is fine, Kev. Just sign the card 'Love, John', and have them delivered to her. I don't have money to give you now, but I'll give it to you when I get back home."

The next day I went to the flower shop and picked out a plant. I signed the card, 'Love, John'.

Eight years later, that plant still blooms.

• • •

On Wednesday of the following week we were provided with some encouraging news. Based on their examinations, the doctors felt confident that the steroids were helping to control the tumors. Also, the mark on Dad's adrenal gland hadn't shown any growth, and the doctors were now hopeful that it wasn't another tumor.

The plan now was to take Dad off the steroids for a rest period while he continued radiation. They would take another CATSCAN in six weeks to see if the tumors had shrunk. It was Dad's choice whether to stay in the hospital or go home. He chose home.

The six weeks was encouraging. It was like a guarantee that he would live at least six more weeks. The immediate urgency we had felt for several days was somewhat lifted. And even better, Dad could come home.

But the encouraging news and the six weeks were false hope. Dad survived only three more weeks and he never felt well again. He had painkillers and some other medicines he could take, but they never made him feel well enough to be very happy. Yet he did not turn into the grouchy, moody person that the nurses warned us about. They said we wouldn't know him, that he would be mean and nasty to everyone because that's how people get when they think they are being cheated out of life. But he never got like that. He accepted the cards that had been dealt to him, and he prayed that somehow, he would be able to get through it.

He underwent intense radiation five days a week. Mom drove him to the hospital each day. On the ride down they held hands and prayed together. They prayed for a miracle.

One day at the hospital while Dad was undergoing radiation, a nurse said something tasteless to Mom. "Soon, he won't even know you," she told Mom. She was referring to the effect that the brain cancer would have on his memory.

Mom ignored the woman. It was bad enough her soul mate was slipping away. She would miss his warmth, his kind heart, the romance they had together. She would miss the advice he had for any situation. She would miss out on the trips they were going to take in their retirement years. She would miss seeing him with their grandchildren. She would miss their 35th wedding anniversary. She would miss growing old with him.

Physically, Dad did change a bit. The radiation was strong and it was centered directly on his head. For the first time, his hair began to fall out, though my plans to shave my head didn't seem appropriate anymore. He also developed a nasty rash on the right side of his face from the exposure. And he lost even more weight, and was looking disgustingly thin.

The radiation greatly affected his energy level. During the weekdays when I was at school, I talked to Mom, and to Dad when he was up to it. Both of them told me how poorly he was feeling and that he had no energy at all. Each weekend when I saw him, though, he seemed to be better than what was described to me on the phone.

I thought maybe I was producing that result, so I made sure I got home as early as possible each weekend. But it wasn't me; it was the fact that he had no radiation on the weekends that made him feel stronger, especially on Sunday after two days of rest. I can only imagine how much he dreaded going back for the radiation every Monday.

•   •   •

Dad spent most of his three weeks at home on the couch in the living room. When he woke from a nap, my mother would sit next to him and he would place his head on her shoulders. Make it go away, his body language suggested. She would hold him there until he went back to lying down. She wished there was more she could do.

Dad slept a lot and watched some television. He wasn't well enough to do any reading. I came home every Friday night and stayed each time until Monday morning. He'd talk to me a little bit whenever he felt well. For the most part, however, he just lay there, surviving, saying his *Our Fathers* and praying for a miracle.

During the week, he was taken care of by my mother in the morning—an aide also came by in the mornings to check on him and help him out—my sister in the afternoon, my brother Patrick when he could, and our dog, Jojo the boxer, all the time.

Dad had a funny affection for Jojo. It was as if he loved her, just as he loved the rest of us. He accepted her as family. When she was a puppy, they had battles. Dad tried to confine her to a small space so that she didn't have the run of the house when we weren't home, but the dog seemed to win all the time. No matter what obstacle he put up, she broke through it. One time, he decided to put her in the washer room and close the door. The door had tiny slats on it and she broke two of them and had fun roaming the house while we were out. Eventually, we bought a cage to put her in when nobody was home, and after she outgrew her little puppy stage and earned some trust, Dad allowed her the run of the house. When it came to playing, however,

Jojo was always a puppy. She used to drop sticks and balls in front of the mower and Dad would have to get off the mower and pick them up. Sometimes he'd throw them for her as if to play, and sometimes he'd hurl them away deep into the woods, thinking she would never find them. But no matter how far he threw her toys and sticks, Jojo chased them and brought them back every time, even blue racquetballs when it was pitch dark out. Eventually, Dad learned ways to make it easier on him to play with her. He would fake a long throw while throwing the ball only a few feet, and those were harder for her to find because she immediately ran into the woods and started sniffing. One day he told me "I found a way to get Jojo tired faster." He threw the ball up the hill so that she would have to run uphill each time. Then he only had to make half as many throws before she would get tired and leave him alone. He got a kick out of the way her tiny stub of a tail would wag when he called her name in a high-pitched voice. Sometimes, when I wasn't home for her to sleep with, Dad would wake up in the middle of the night to find that Jojo had stolen his covers and was lying on them on the floor.

But during the three weeks Dad was home, Jojo lay by his side the whole time. She knew he wasn't well. She never asked him to let her outside or to play with her. She just laid her body against the couch, trying to get as close to him as she could.

When walking through my parents' room one day six months later, Jojo picked up his scent on a piece of clothing and began to whimper. Even she knew he was special.

• • •

One Sunday during the three weeks Dad was home, he sat down for a nice dinner with the family. He tried to eat, but couldn't manage more than a few bites, yet he stayed at the table and talked with us for a while before having to excuse himself. Then he went into the living room to lie down.

A few minutes later, I went inside to talk to him. I asked how he was feeling and he smiled at me. That was his way during those weeks. It was quite an effort for him to talk, so usually he just smiled.

As I was sitting there, Jamie and Benjamin came into the room. "Are you watching this, Grandpa?" Jamie asked as she pointed to the television. It was tuned to a news show, with the audio very low.

"Yes," Dad said softly.

The kids began walking down the stairs, but Dad shouted after them. "Jamie! Benjamin!"

His voice couldn't project very far. It made me cringe to hear him yell. It was such an effort. I walked over to the stairs and yelled, "Jamie! Benjamin! Grandpa wants you!" They came back up the stairs.

"Do you guys want to watch something?" Dad asked them.

Jamie nodded her head. "We can watch it downstairs though, it's okay, Grandpa."

"No, you can watch it up here if you want. Is that okay with you, Kev?"

Okay with me?

I couldn't believe it. He felt so poorly. He tried to eat dinner and he couldn't. He sat at the table and talked to us for a while until his energy had been spent. He had to excuse himself from the table and go inside to lie down. He played the television only softly, and when I came into the room he could barely even manage a smile. But he shouted as loud as he could to tell his grandchildren they could watch television in the living room. He knew he was subjecting himself to a loud television and lots of laughing over the next hour, but he just wanted to be near them. His revere for other people was amazing. He loved his grandchildren. He wanted to see them grow up. They were one of the reasons he was fighting so hard to stay alive.

• • •

Dad began losing his patience with food. He couldn't eat anything. If he didn't eat one thing, we'd suggest something else. I didn't know what could make him well, but I did know that if he didn't start eating more, he would certainly die. One night I tried to reach out to him as delicately as I could. I spoke to him and Mom in the living room.

"You know how some people feel that their dog is the best dog in the world? And no matter what you say about your own dog, and how special it is, they will never concede that your dog is better than theirs?"

Dad smiled at me and nodded his head.

"Well, that's how I feel about you guys. I think that nobody beats my mother and father."

Dad smiled. I could see he wanted to cry, but he didn't have the energy. I walked over to him.

"I know it's tough, Dad. I can't imagine how tough. But we want you to get better," I told him as I reached back to Mom. "We think you can do it. But we know you'll *never* get better unless you start eating."

He nodded. "I'll try, Kev," he said to me softly. I hugged him. Mom came over and hugged us both.

That was one of the few times in my life when I felt I was in a position to point out something he failed to see. I thought maybe he needed a little kick to get him going, just as I had needed one a number of times and he had delivered. I couldn't live with myself if I didn't try. But he didn't need a kick. I just could not comprehend the extent to which his suffering had grown, and I was running out of ideas on how to help. I grasped at anything during this time; an article in the newspaper about a boy in Texas going for experimental brain cancer treatment; a hint of hope in the doctor's words; a smile from Dad.

But I couldn't fix his brain. I couldn't pull out the tumors. I couldn't rescue him. I was helpless.

• • •

A social worker came to the house one day during the three weeks Dad was home. Dad didn't want to see her at first, but after she left, he was glad she had come. Her name was Joanne.

"Is there anything on your mind that you would like to get out into the open?" Joanne asked.

Silence.

"Either one of you?"

Silence.

"Anything at all?"

"Well," Dad finally spoke, "I have a lot of tools from the woodcarving club that I sell. Warren tools. I don't think anyone will know how much they're worth."

"You can do something about that," Joanne told him. "Is that it?"

Dad looked at Mom and held her hand. "Yeah, I think that's it."

"Silence is good," Joanne told them.

It was Joanne's experience that people who were not fulfilled in their lives usually took that opportunity to express their love, or to apologize, or tell secrets that they had kept. They normally said things like "I want my kids to know I love them" and express regret over things they did or never got to do. But when people didn't take the opportunity to talk about these things, it meant they were fulfilled in their lives.

I wondered what was going through Dad's mind when he wrote a price list for the tools the next weekend. He took his time going over the list and checking the prices. He made sure it was exactly right. He made sure it was neat. Yet he knew the list would only be used in the event of his death.

• • •

During the weeks of his struggle with brain cancer, my father asked not to see anyone except his wife and children. That even included Mr. Littmann, who called almost every day to ask how Dad was feeling and if he was up to a visitor or a telephone conversation. After he learned of the brain cancer, however, Dad never entertained another guest.

My father was a strong man. He was dignified and proud. He would not allow any guest to come to his house and see him lying on the couch. That would have embarrassed him. It would have made it look as if the cancer had beaten him, and that would not have accurately described the toughness with which he had fought it. For his friends to see him at that time would have misrepresented all that he was and all he had fought so hard to hold onto.

Had anyone come to the house during that period, he would have had to expend all his energy in entertaining them, for he would not have lain on the couch and let people feel bad for him. He was the kind of person who commanded respect, not sympathy. He had raised a family, built a home, and had a successful career. He read books, built things, fixed stuff, and earned the respect of everyone he knew.

And he was going to be healthy again. He wanted to see all of his friends, and his nieces and nephews too, but he wanted to see them after he recovered. If he were going to get through this, it would be through his strength and the strength of his wife and children and the realization that others were thinking of him and praying for him. For others to see him in his weakened state would have had a negative effect on his recovery. What kept him strong was the fact that he knew that when he recovered, others would see him as the man they always knew, and as a man who was too strong to let a disease defeat him.

I asked him one day, half seriously, if he was interested in looking into an experimental treatment that a hospital in Texas was doing for brain cancer patients. I'm not sure if he would have fit in with their program anyway, but it would have meant flying him to Texas. He shook his head at the idea. He just wanted the cancer to go away. He had no energy left for something like that. He had outlasted the chemotherapy and the radiation. He had fought the cancer and survived the surgery. Then, when he should have begun to recover, there had been another surgery to contend with. He handled that. And he had enough left to go through that recovery. But he had saved no energy for what was happening to him now.

It was as if he had entered a one mile race and won, only to find out at the finish line, when his energy was exhausted, that it had been changed to a five mile race, and upon winning that one, to a marathon. Part of him must have felt bitter, even cheated, and if he did, he was no different from any of his family, or from others who have gone through something similar. He had fought so hard to keep his life. But he also knew, as he had once said to me, that what was happening to him was part of life.

Dad chose to spend what was left of his energy at home, praying that he would get better. And if he didn't get better, at least he knew he was spending his last bit of time in the house he had built, where his family had grown up. He would spend the time with his wife, constantly reminded of his greatest accomplishment in life.

• • •

It was a Friday. I was hitting racquetballs at the school gym seventy miles away. I was planning to go to work later that day, then drive upstate to see Dad and spend the weekend with him.

In the locker room following my workout, I heard a quick, single beep coming from my pager. Someone had tried to reach me while I was on the court.

My pants were hanging from a hook in my locker and I reached into the right pocket for the beeper. The number on the display screen was Dianne's, with a nine following the seven digit number. It could mean that she meant to press 911, indicating that it was urgent. It could also mean that she punched in her number and accidentally hit nine afterwards. The time on the page was 12:58, an hour old, so I figured that it could probably wait a few more minutes until after I changed.

I thought about Dad as I sat on the bench. His radiation treatments had ended three days earlier, and I was excited that his energy level might increase. When he was going to bed the previous Sunday, I had said to him, "Just try to get through these next two days, Dad. They're the last two days of radiation, then your body can begin to recuperate and you'll feel strong again."

The treatments were having such a hard effect on his body. It was as though he was an automobile and we were the drivers. The car was going uphill and riding on fumes from an empty gas tank, but we figured that if the car could get over the crest, there was bound to be a downhill on the other side. And if we caught a break, there just might be a gas station we could coast to. I honestly felt that he had a chance at recovery if he could get through those two days.

He nodded slowly and said, "See you next week...maybe." while shaking his head.

What did he mean by *maybe*, I thought to myself. It may have been his way of saying to me that I wasn't obligated to be there next weekend and that if it were too much for me to make it home, he would understand.

"Oh, I'll definitely be home next weekend, don't worry about that," I told him.

He nodded again.

"Can I help you get your legs onto the bed?"

"I'm not ready yet, besides, I can manage it myself."

"Okay, Dad."

As I walked towards the door I heard him say, "I love you."

"I love *you*, Dad," I told him.

Had I known what would happen that next week, I would have thought of something more to say.

Before I left for Long Island the next morning, I went into my parents' room and saw Dad cuddled with Mom in bed. I wanted Mom to know I was leaving and she didn't need to wake me. She was asleep, but Dad opened his eyes. I stuck my thumb up and silently mouthed "I'm going." He nodded his head just enough to indicate that he understood and I needn't wake Mom. Then he gave me one of his smiles.

I talked to him once more on Wednesday. I called Sharon and asked her to go upstairs and tell Dad I called and that if he felt up to talking, I was at work and not too busy.

"I'll tell him," Sharon said, "but I wouldn't expect a call back. He's really feeling poorly."

Five minutes later, though, he was on the phone talking to me. I congratulated him on finishing the radiation, although he said he was disappointed that he didn't feel any better yet.

"I'm looking forward to seeing you this weekend. You should rest until then so that you feel better for our meeting."

"Okay," he said.

I never heard his voice again.

• • •

Sharon had a long talk with Dad the night before he died. She said that she told him to get better, and although he had been responding to statements like that by saying, "I'll try," he responded that time by saying, "Tomorrow. I'm going to get better tomorrow."

Mom came home to find him in a strange position on the bed that night. Sharon had offered to help him into bed earlier but he had told her he could manage. Apparently, though, he did not have enough strength to lift his legs completely onto the bed. Mom found him with his legs hanging half off the bed. She heard him say he felt that maybe he should be in a hospital. He was still fighting hard for his life, because if he had given up and thought he was going to die, he would have wanted to be at home.

I don't really believe people are forewarned of their death with any certainty. If they were, I imagine there would be more tears and long goodbyes, and other things that would be talked about. I think it is just that these last acts get magnified and over-analyzed simply because they *are* the last acts of a person, and the "do you think he or she knew?" question always seems to surface. But without hindsight, it was just another day.

• • •

I was hungry as I was leaving the locker room but I figured I should call Dianne before getting lunch. I stopped at the pay phone in the gymnasium to call. Dianne picked up on the fourth ring. "Hello."

"Hi Dianne."

"Kev, where are you?" I feared where-are-yous.

"I'm at the school, I just finished my workout."

"Oooooooooh Kev," she said in a sympathetic voice.

"What?"

"Bad news," she said.

Dad didn't even come to mind. I so badly wanted to believe it was something else.

"It's Dad. He's gone, Kev."

Thoughts rushed through my head. Dianne must be mistaken. He can't be gone yet. Wait, maybe she meant the cancer was gone. No, okay, then surely the doctors were having a pressure packed day and misinterpreted Dad's vital signs. Give it another try doctors, you're wrong! He's not dead! How can I reach them before it's too late? How can I get them to resuscitate him? Try again!

"I'm so sorry, Kevin," Dianne said. "Why don't you come here?"

"Okay. I'll come soon."

I hung up the phone and stared at it. I look at the ceiling, then back at the phone. I folded my arms, and then unfolded them. I picked up the receiver and slammed it down as hard as I could! I picked up the receiver again, and slammed it down…hard! I slammed it again and again! I hoped that some guy would walk by and object to my slamming the phone so I could close my fist and take a shot at him. I'll lay him out on the floor and watch him suffer in pain, and enjoy every second of it! You'll suffer!

Instead of finding someone to hit, I walked to my car, drove for a while, stopped for a hamburger, and went to Dianne's. From there I called Mom, who sounded pretty together for what she had been through.

● ● ●

There are some details surrounding my father's illness and death in which it is not clear exactly what happened. Where did he really die? Did the doctors do everything they could, or could they have done more? Since nothing will change the outcome of my father's death, I choose to believe the versions that comfort me the most. I think it is the right thing to do when remembering someone, and I would recommend it for all those who have lost loved ones. There is nothing more you can do for the person. Life is for the living. You must do whatever you can for yourself.

So what I believe happened is what happened. Nobody can convince me of anything else. And nobody can convince me that there isn't a God and a special place where special people go. They don't just fade away.

When my father woke that morning, God had already made his decision and there was nothing that could have prevented what happened. Around 10:15, the aide who had been coming to the house yelled to my mother in the kitchen that she needed help with Dad. Mom had already helped Dad get from the bed to the bathroom. In a very weak voice he told her, "I can't do this anymore". None of us are sure what he meant by that.

Together, the two women began helping Dad off the toilet and back to bed, but he never made it out of the bathroom. He collapsed onto the floor. Mom called 911 and the aide began yelling in his ear as she had been taught to do. As they waited for the paramedics to arrive, my mother sat on the cold bathroom floor, holding my father in her arms.

The doctors said that Dad might have been suffering more than anybody knew. He had complained during the last week of pains in his chest and stomach areas. When Mom showed the doctors where Dad had complained of pain, they told her that it was not near the adrenal gland. They now felt the cancer might have spread all over Dad's body. Maybe we were lucky that he died that day rather than live another few weeks. During those weeks, the pain would have become unbearable, and the cancer in his brain would have robbed him of his memory.

There was a story that surfaced some months after my father's death about what happened after the paramedics arrived. It had something to do with a neighbor who had a friend whose daughter dated a cop. The cop said he talked to a nurse at Arden Hill who knew the nurse that was in the emergency room with my father when they brought him in. That nurse, now six sources removed, supposedly said that Dad was still alive when he was brought into the emergency room, and that he told her not to let his wife see him the way he was. I think the whole circle was just a bunch of people looking for something to whisper about, something they thought they knew that nobody else did. The truth is, had he been alive at that point, there is no way he would have been able to communicate to anyone what was going through his mind. I don't believe any part of that story.

What I do believe is based on my faith and on what my mother has told me. The official death certificate reads that Dad died at Arden Hill Hospital in Goshen. But that is not true. His soul had left this earth before the paramedics arrived at the house. My father's last moments on earth were spent in the arms of my mother. As she sat on the cold bathroom floor holding him on that Friday morning in

March, Jesus came from heaven and put His arms underneath hers and lifted Dad away with Him.

He passed directly from Mom to God. There was nothing in between.

Our Last Promise

The week before his last Father's Day, I told Dad I wanted to take him fishing at the stream, the stream where Mom once told me he went to relieve stress and dream a little.

"Fishing?" he said with a bright smile. "We haven't been fishing in many years. Yeah, that would be fun."

The night before Father's Day, I called Dad at midnight to say I wouldn't get home until six the next morning, and although I was willing to stay awake and go fishing, Dad said, "I'd rather see you get some sleep. We'll make plans to go another time. It doesn't have to be on Father's Day."

We put it off until late in the summer, but by then, he was feeling too sick to go, though he had not yet been diagnosed with cancer. So we made a promise that we would go fishing the following Father's Day, with no excuses allowed.

The next Father's Day, I returned to the stream; however, I was alone. I didn't fish. I just sat on the rocks and listened to the crisp sounds of water trickling down the slope, remembering the first time I was there as a kid, when

Mom was feeling overwhelmed with life and Dad sat underneath the big oak tree and comforted her.

I looked to see if he would return to this place now to keep his end of our promise. I looked for him to be standing on a center rock, gracefully swaying the line from side to side, then easing it into the water. I waited patiently for hours for him to appear, waiting for a sign from God, for some form of magic from the afterworld to take effect and bring him back, even if for just a moment. But nothing happened.

Dad was unable to keep our last promise, but as the water splashed against the rock on which I sat, I heard his voice inside my head reminding me, "It's part of life, Kev."

He did, however, leave behind his spirit and I found part of that spirit at the fishing stream that Father's Day. As the years have passed, I've learned to call on that spirit when I have needed it most.

Recommend me to a friend

Are you looking for a gift for a friend?

Did you borrow this book from a friend or library?

For copies of Our *Last Promise*, check your local bookstore or order autographed copies through this form.

Please send me ＿＿ autographed copies at $14.95 each
Please send me ＿＿ non-autographed copies at $14.95 each

Include $3.50 shipping and handling. New York residents must include applicable sales tax. Canadian order must include payment in USD. All payments must accompany order.

＿＿ My check or money order for $＿＿＿ is enclosed
＿＿ Please charge my ＿＿ Visa ＿＿ Mastercard

Name ＿＿＿＿＿＿＿＿＿＿＿＿＿＿＿＿＿＿＿＿＿

Address ＿＿＿＿＿＿＿＿＿＿＿＿＿＿＿＿＿＿＿

City/State/Zip ＿＿＿＿＿＿＿＿＿＿＿＿＿＿＿＿

Phone ＿＿＿＿＿＿＿＿＿＿ Email＿＿＿＿＿＿＿

Card # ＿＿＿＿＿＿＿＿＿＿＿＿＿＿＿＿＿＿＿

Exp Date ＿＿＿＿＿＿ Signature ＿＿＿＿＿＿＿

Make your check payable to:
Blue Hudson Publishing
72-11 Austin Street #190, Forest Hills, NY 11375

OR CALL 1-800-781-7595
OR ORDER ON THE WEB AT
www.ourlastpromise.com

Please check our web site at

www.bluehudson.com

for information on:
Fundraising for charities and groups
Additional books
Articles
"Writing Away the Pain" workshops

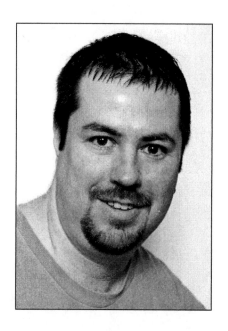

About the Author

Kevin Murphy lives in Kew Gardens, NY. He is the founder of the "Writing Away the Pain" workshops.